THE FAT LADY HASN'T SUNG
An Inspiring Story of Love, Hope and Triumph

THE FAT LADY HASN'T SUNG

An Inspiring Story of Love, Hope, and Triumph

BY MARY WALKER

Hill Country Books
San Antonio, Texas

THE FAT LADY HASN'T SUNG

An Inspiring Story of Love, Hope, and Triumph

BY MARY WALKER

Published by: Hill Country Books
              Post Office Box 791615
              San Antonio, TX 78279-1615 U.S.A.

Copyright © 1995 by Mary C. Walker. All rights reserved. The contents and cover design are protected by copyright. No part of this book may be reproduced in any form without permission in writing from the publisher, except for a reviewer who wishes to quote brief passages in connection with a review written for inclusion in a magazine or newspaper.

Printed in the United States of America

Cover design by Robert E. Gilley, Ft. Worth

Library of Congress Catalog Card Number: 94-96713

Publisher's Cataloging in Publication Data
Walker, Mary C., 1936-
The Fat Lady Hasn't Sung: An Inspiring Story of Love, Hope, and
    Triumph/by Mary Walker
312p. 22cm.
1. Walker, Mary, 1936-   –Health. 2. Cancer–Patients–United
    States–Biography. I. Title.
RC280.B8W35 1995
362.196994490092 W177
ISBN 0-9644374-6-5: $14.95 Softcover

To Jack:

*My husband, my lover, and my best friend.
With his love, help, and
understanding,
anything is
possible.*

The story you are about to read is true. I have changed the names of several persons to maintain the anonymity of the innocent and to protect the guilty!

—Mary Walker

Chapter One

The flashing lights in my rearview mirror were unmistakably those of a police car. As I pulled over to the shoulder of the freeway, I knew I would have a tough time explaining what was going on.

I had been shopping on my usual Friday rounds in San Antonio. It seems everything was going *too* smoothly that day, even though it was unseasonably cold and windy. My electric wheelchair had operated flawlessly. My lift van had responded perfectly during my many stops. And my husband, Jack, wouldn't believe that I was going to be home at our prearranged time.

I don't usually set a specific time to be home (because of my dependency on mechanical devices), but this particular weekend we were going to the Houston Grand Opera to hear Verdi's *Otello* with Placido Domingo. (Jack has been an opera lover most of his life, and, with infinite patience, he has taught me to love this beautiful art form as well).

Then it happened! At my last scheduled stop at the grocery store, I couldn't close the lift mechanism on my van.

My lift van, a converted Dodge Caravan, is my pride and joy

since it is my key to independence. Due to its cost, Jack jokingly refers to it as "Mary's Mercedes" in a Dodge body.

It is quite a remarkable machine. When the van is closed, I can open it from the outside by turning a key. This causes the rear door to open and rise straight up, resembling the mouth of the shark, "Jaws." The heavy steel mesh ramp flops down to a horizontal position, extending out from the rear about four feet. It then slowly lowers to ground level. I can then maneuver my chair onto the ramp. By flipping a switch, the process is reversed; my wheelchair is lifted aboard, and the rear door closes securely just like the whale swallowing Jonah.

Once inside, I transfer to the driver's seat and move it to the proper position. When driving, hand controls allow me to accelerate or brake. When I operate the van, it is rare not to have an audience of admiring spectators.

On this Friday, the young man carrying out my groceries was up to his usual good-natured small talk about my van. "I guess we're gonna have 'show time' again today, huh, Mrs. Walker?"

"Let's hope so. We both want to get out of this cold wind," I replied.

But today was to be different. After loading myself and my groceries, I pushed the switch to close the ramp and rear door. Nothing happened! After numerous attempts to close the van, I was still left with my "runway down."

By this time a small crowd had assembled to help. The parking lot consultants' suggestions proved to be futile.

Glancing at my watch, I knew it was too late to call Jack at his office since he would be on his way home. So, I decided my only choice was to attempt to get to the van repair shop before closing time. As I drove out of the parking lot with my rear door up and my ramp out, I realized I had less than 30 minutes.

My heart sank as I saw the police officer emerge from his car with ticket book in hand. He was a typical Texan—tall, lanky, and, at this moment, seemed larger than life.

"Ma'm, do you realize your rear door is open and something is stickin' out from this van?" he drawled as he arranged the carbon paper in his book.

"I may be numb from the cold, but I'm not blind," I laughed, trying to inject a humorous note in an otherwise embarrassing situation.

"You'll have to get out of the car and show me your driver's license," he grunted as my attempt at humor obviously fell on deaf ears.

"Well, officer, therein lies the rub." His face looked blank. I began to explain that I couldn't stand, walk, or even use crutches. I told him that I was confined to a wheelchair, that my van lift had suffered a mechanical failure, and I now had less than ten minutes to get to the shop before closing.

"Well, little lady, you just follow me, and we'll get you to the shop on time," he smiled as his mood visibly changed from hostility to helpfulness.

With his flashing lights ahead of me and his siren wailing, we zipped down McAllister Freeway with traffic pulling to the left and right like the Red Sea parting before Moses.

Chapter Two

My life has not always been so inextricably bound to the wheel.

The spring and early summer of 1973 had been reasonably pleasant for Jack and me. Our two children, David, 7, and Amy, 5, had finally become independent swimmers—that is, they were able to jump in the water and swim, mostly under water like tadpoles, for considerable distances without assistance. I guess my efforts at making them water babies as infants finally was paying off.

I had learned to swim at an early age at the "cesspool" (my grandmother's term for the city swimming pool) in my hometown of Estherville, Iowa. After many years of living with swimmer's ear and chlorine-red eyes, I became proficient enough to swim professionally for four summers with the Aqua Follies, a synchronized swimming group of 24 swimmers who performed as part of the Minneapolis Aquatennial.

In addition to numerous performances in Minneapolis, we traveled to Seattle and Detroit each summer to perform in their annual water festivals. I also taught swimming to youngsters during the summer months of my college years at Lake Calhoun in Minneapolis. This job became available to me because I was a physical education major at Mankato State College in Minnesota.

During that time I observed children who were literally petrified from fear of water. I almost lost part of my anatomy one July day to a six-year old boy who honestly believed his life would be at stake if he were to loosen his grip on me for even an instant. Therefore, I was determined that my own children would be exposed to water in a natural way at the earliest possible age.

As a daily routine the children and I would make our afternoon trek to our community pool in Rockville, Maryland, a suburb of Washington, D.C.

Jack and I had purchased our first home the year before after Jack had been transferred by the Navy from Guam to Washington, D.C. We loved our Rockville home—a typical center-hall, two-story colonial—because it was ideal for our family. It was situated on a quiet cul-de-sac, and it had a finished, walk-out basement which immediately became a play room for the children.

It was during these trips to the pool—about a quarter of a mile each way—that I first noticed I was having some difficulties walking. One afternoon as Jack was coming home from work he noticed the three of us trudging home hot and tired from our afternoon swim. He stopped his car near us.

"Last one home has to wash the dishes," he yelled.

By the time he followed the road around to the front of our house, the kids already were home and waiting. Jack parked his car in the garage and got out. He looked cool in his summer white Navy Commander's uniform.

"Mom's got to wash dishes tonight," the kids cheered.

"Looks that way," he laughed, as I approached them.

Jack greeted me with his customary kiss.

"Why are you limping, Honey?" he asked with concern.

"I didn't know I was. Maybe it's old age," I replied since I was going to be 37 in September.

"You'd better have that checked again," he warned. "You're developing an orthopedic limp."

My first indication of a problem with my leg occurred in May of 1973. Jack and I had been to a surprise birthday party for our good friend, Dow Berggren, planned by his wife, Debbie. Jack and Dow had first met in 1954 at Newport, Rhode Island, where they were completing Navy Officer Candidate School. After graduation from OCS, they were ordered to Washington, D.C. for duty. Jack, Dow, and two other bachelor Navy ensigns rented a town house in Alexandria, Virginia, where they lived for the first two years of their Naval careers.

After a superb evening with many old friends, Jack and I returned home around midnight, paid our baby sitter, and were fast asleep by 12:30 a.m. Shortly after 3 a.m., I awoke suddenly with a sharp, excruciating pain in my left thigh. I sat bolt upright in bed, moaning softly. I had never felt any pain like that before. Jack, who has always been a light sleeper, awoke as I sat up.

"What's wrong?" he asked in a sleepy, thick-tongued voice.

"I don't know. It's either a cramp or a charley horse."

"Is there anything I can do?"

"No, thanks. I think I'll try to walk it out," I whispered as I got out of bed and started walking around our bedroom.

After about 15 minutes of walking and rubbing my leg, I took a couple of aspirins and went back to bed. Since I wasn't used to taking any pain medication, the aspirins worked their magic, and I finally drifted back to sleep.

When we got up later that morning, my leg was still sore, but it wasn't that sharp, piercing pain that had awakened me from a sound sleep. Besides, Judy Husebo, my high school friend from Minneapolis, was coming over to spend the day with us. And I didn't have time to worry about some silly old pain.

By mid-week, at Jack's persistence, I reluctantly reported to orthopedic "walk-in" at Bethesda Naval Hospital. Walk-in clinic is designed for patients with minor complaints which can be treated on an out-patient basis. Patients are handled on a priority basis depending on the severity of the problem. Since I appeared relatively normal (I didn't have any broken bones protruding through my skin), I was relegated to low man on the totem pole to see a doctor.

After what seemed to be an interminable wait, a young doctor poked his head around the corner of the room and called my name. As we sat in his cubical of an office, he introduced himself and asked the inevitable question.

"I'm Dr. Allen. What seems to be the problem today?"

I told him about the pain attack early last Sunday and the subsequent soreness.

"Well, hop up on the table, and we'll take a look."

He proceeded to check my range of motion, reflexes, and nerve responses in both legs.

"Everything appears okay from what I can see. But since I'm not Superman with X-ray vision, we're going to have to take some pictures," he added, as he scribbled on an X-ray form.

I hurried down the hall to the X-ray area and caught the technician just as he was about to take his lunch break.

"I bet you're on your way to the mess hall."

"As a matter of fact, I'm dining at McDonald's for lunch," he replied as he scanned the request form. "These won't take long to shoot."

As I get older medical people seem to get younger and younger. My X-ray technician was no exception. He was a tall, thin, seraphic young man of about 19. His smooth, pink cheeks were crowned with a head of straight blond hair, cut in bangs over his forehead.

"Okay, Mrs. Walker, I need you to frog leg."

"Frog leg?" I asked incredulously. "Do you want me to demonstrate in a pool?"

"No, just do your Kermit the Frog imitation on the table."

If I hadn't known before that he was young, he confirmed it with that reference to "Sesame Street." Thank goodness I had become familiar with Kermit and his friends by watching the show with David and Amy.

Armed with my frog leg pictures, along with several other

views of my body in positions I didn't know I could get into, I returned to Dr. Allen's office.

"I don't see anything abnormal," he mumbled as he looked intently at the X-rays on his viewer. "My best guess is that you've pulled a muscle. I'm going to send you to physical therapy for diathermy treatments."

Although I was relieved to hear that the X-rays were normal, I wondered how on earth I could have pulled a muscle while lying in bed.

Chapter Three

"Mrs. Walker," the voice rang out unemotionally.

"Here I am, Dr. Allen. I'm just like a bad penny—I keep turning up," I smiled as I followed him into his cubicle.

As we exchanged pleasantries, I noticed more than ever before that his face was cast in a perpetually bored expression. Dr. Allen was a short man of about 30 with dark, piercing eyes and a thin smile.

"Well, the physical therapy didn't work," I began. "If anything, I'm worse now than I was before. And to quote my husband, I've developed an orthopedic limp."

Dr. Allen sat silently as he flipped through the pages of my medical record, refreshing his memory of my previous visit. After a long silence, he wrinkled his brow and drew a deep breath: "I think I'll send you to rheumatology. Maybe this is an arthritic condition."

While military medicine in general is excellent, there are peripheral nuisances associated with such large-scale health delivery systems. One such persistent problem is obtaining routine appointments. My referral by Dr. Allen to the rheumatology clinic was typical. The first available opening was in late August.

As I reported for my appointment, I was met by the stereotypical military hospital appointment clerk: a self-important, late middle-aged old crone who jealousy protects the physicians' time like Fafner guarding the Nibelung hoard.

After a brief wait, a tall, well-built man of about 35 approached me and introduced himself. Dr. Jackson then led me into his spacious office.

"I see by the referral that you've developed a limp, Mrs. Walker. Why don't you tell me how all this happened?"

I recounted to Dr. Jackson the chronology of my problem since May.

After a typical orthopedic exam, Dr. Jackson began to fill out what seemed like dozens of forms.

"I want you to complete all this blood work before I see you again next month," he instructed. He was requesting sedimentation rates, complete blood count, and uric acid levels among other items on the various slips of paper.

Observing my worried look, he asked: "Is there a problem?"

"I don't believe I'll be able to see you next month. I'm having a hysterectomy the second week of September."

My history of "female problems" went back a long way. It would be hard to pinpoint the exact date of my first female difficulty. However, by the time Jack and I had been married four years, I had experienced an ectopic pregnancy and a uterine suspension. Since I was still having problems, Dr. Norris, my current gynecologist, recommended a complete hysterectomy.

"That's no problem," Dr. Jackson reassured me. "Come back to see me in October. In the meantime, I'll prescribe some anti-inflammatory drugs to help your leg."

My hysterectomy was timed to coincide with the beginning of school. Amy was starting first grade, and it would be easier for Jack to ride herd on the children during my hospital stay because they would both be in school for the full day. My mother, Mildred Crawford, planned to arrive to help out after my return home from the hospital.

The Fat Lady Hasn't Sung

The night before my surgery, Dr. Norris breezed into my hospital room at Bethesda with a consent form. As is customary in military hospitals, he launched into a litany of the possible risks and outcomes from such medical procedures, up to and including death.

Dr. Norris had an intent look about him as he peered at me through his wire-rimmed glasses. I thought to myself that his hair style was about 20 years out of fashion as I observed his greased-down "duck tails."

"Now this surgery should be fairly routine. We don't expect any surprises. It shouldn't take more than about two hours. Tell your husband I'll meet him back here in your room afterward to let him know how it went."

After Dr. Norris said goodbye, I had my first chance to look around the GYN ward of Bethesda Naval Hospital.

Military hospitals vary tremendously in their privacy and amenities for patients.

Rodriguez Army Hospital in Puerto Rico provided my first exposure to military hospitals. It was there in 1961 that my left Fallopian tube had been removed due to my ectopic pregnancy. Within view of the hospital was El Morro Castle with its weathered stone walls and ancient lookout towers. The OB-GYN ward at Rodriguez was housed in the main hospital building. It reminded me of an old Spanish convent with its thick walls and high ceilings. Row upon row of white hospital beds stretched across vast stone floors. Since there was no air conditioning, the huge windows were perpetually open, catching the humid Caribbean Sea breezes. As charming as these old buildings were, their venerable construction style precluded the use of certain modern electronic conveniences. For example, instead of pushing a button to "call" for a nurse, a patient had to have a loud voice or be able to whistle through his teeth. Fortunately, I learned to do the latter when I was a seventh grader. (I paid a price of three days in detention hall for acquiring this skill since my first successful whistle was produced one afternoon in study hall).

My next experience in a military hospital was in 1963 in Bremerhaven, Germany. The U.S. Army Hospital was housed in a building that had served as a hospital for the Third Reich. Although the swastika had been removed, the Nazi German eagle symbol was still in place above the front entry. There were other, more subtle, relics of Germany's Nazi past throughout the hospital. Kurt Schultz was one of the civilian employees from the admissions office. He was a tall, slender man in his late forties who prided himself on his efficiency. Even without a monocle, his physical appearance mirrored the Hollywood image of a Nazi officer. I would tease Jack by threatening to sneak up behind Herr Schultz and yell *"Sieg Heil!"* Although I never got up enough nerve to do it, Jack and I both agreed that Herr Schultz would automatically snap to attention and click his leather boot heels together.

Thanks in part to Herr Schultz's managerial prowess, coupled with a temporary shortfall in patients, I was assigned to a lovely, private room, complete with an electronic call system.

After fully recovering from my earlier ectopic pregnancy in Puerto Rico, my gynecologist in Bremerhaven informed me that I had a "tipped" uterus. Such a condition, he assured me, would prevent successful future pregnancies. He recommended that I undergo a surgical procedure called a "uterine suspension." The surgery was uneventful, and my recovery was complete. About the only suspense was whether or not someone would sneak up behind Herr Schultz and bark the magic words.

My accommodations at Bethesda were quite nice. I was assigned to a double room, although the other bed was vacant when I checked in. When I returned from my tour of the GYN ward, the person who was to become my roommate had just arrived. She introduced herself as Barbara Brown. After exchanging pleasantries, we got down to the nitty-gritty.

"Why are you here?" she queried.

"I'm going to have a complete hysterectomy," I replied. "How about you?"

"I'm here for elective surgery," she began. "You know the

kind you need after you've had four kids and your husband starts looking at younger girls more and more. I thought it was time to have things tightened up."

Barbara was quite attractive in a sort of Joan Collins way. Her clothes fit her slender body like a glove. As she changed into her silky bed clothes, I couldn't help noticing that she was wearing matching tiger-striped bikini pants and bra. She saw that I was wearing the traditional government-issue male pajama pants and shirt in men's large size.

"Look at this, Mary. Here's what you need," she gushed as she pulled a Frederick's of Hollywood brochure from her overnight case and pointed out a sexy negligee. "With this outfit you'll have your husband drooling and the doctors waiting in line to see you."

"Well, that's not really me," I laughed. "Normally I wear a football jersey to bed, and Jack says that I'm a frustrated jock."

I knew from her look of disbelief that she couldn't imagine that I really preferred the oversized male pajamas. I changed the subject by saying I was going to turn in early since I was scheduled to be first in the operating room in the morning.

As I drifted off to sleep, Barbara was lying on her bed reading a pulp magazine. The only word I could make out in the title was "Romance."

About an hour and a half after the scheduled starting time for my surgery, Jack told me later that he showed up to wait in my room on the GYN ward as pre-arranged. At the two-hour point, there was no Dr. Norris. Minutes faded into hours. At the three-hour mark, Jack began to pace nervously. The wait had now become agonizing. Four hours had now come and gone. Finally, five hours after the surgery began, Dr. Norris appeared before Jack. His surgical greens were soaked with perspiration, and he looked exhausted both physically and mentally.

Dr. Norris apologized for the long wait and explained that contrary to expectations the surgical team had encountered a big surprise. He said that I had one of the worst cases of endometriosis he had ever seen. Endometriosis, he pointed out, was an abnormal condition in which fragments of the tissue lining the uterus had migrated to other parts of the body and had become implanted there.

I arrived back in my room about dinner time after spending several hours in the recovery room. Shortly after my return, Jack arrived to greet me. He looked tired, but he was smiling.

"How're you feeling?" he asked with a sense of relief. "I've been so worried."

"Fine, I'm just a little groggy at this point. I'm sorry you had to wait so long. I know you were concerned. I can tell by the path you've worn in the floor."

Dr. Norris, still in his greens, popped his head in the door interrupting our conversation.

"I guess your husband told you what we found," he wondered. "It was like a giant spider web. I've never seen anything like it. There was some involvement of the bladder. We had to cut the endometriosis away from it, so your urine will be bloody for several days."

My first visitor the next morning was Dow Berggren. He was his usual ebullient self as he greeted me with a bouquet of flowers. Shortly after Dow's arrival, Jack showed up on his way to work. As we talked, Jack and I began to observe that Dow was becoming increasingly more pale and nervous looking. He had noticed hanging at my bedside a Foley catheter bag which appeared to be filled with blood instead of urine.

After Dow excused himself and said goodbye to me, I closed my eyes for a few seconds. Still visibly shaken, Dow whispered to Jack near my door, thinking he was out of my hearing range.

"Is she going to make it, Jack?"

"Why, sure, of course. The doctor says she'll make a complete recovery. The blood you saw is because they had to do some repair work to her bladder."

Dow looked relieved. I opened my eyes and spoke across the room to the surprised pair: "Jack, Dow looks a little green around the gills. Make sure he's okay before he gets out in that traffic."

My room was like Grand Central Station that day. A parade

of medical specialists came to see Barbara to discuss her upcoming surgery. There were hematologists, cardiologists, urologists, gynecologists, and internal medicine specialists who examined her and discussed her case in great detail. The upshot of all this activity was the conclusion that her dangerously-high blood pressure would make her a surgical risk.

But Barbara felt this surgery was essential to her future happiness and opted to go with it.

I was given the green light earlier that day to walk around the ward, including bathroom privileges. By the time dinner arrived, I was more than ready to get back in bed. Shortly after dinner, I began to feel a nagging pain in my left leg. By bedtime, the pain had grown more intense. I asked the nurse for a couple of aspirins. At midnight, I awoke with an excruciating pain in my left leg, reminiscent of what I had felt the previous May.

I stumbled from my bed carrying my Foley bag and approached the dimly-lit nurses' station.

The Navy nurse behind the desk was a fresh-faced ensign with short, dark hair worn in a page-boy under her crisp, starched cap.

"What are you doing out of bed, Mrs. Walker?" Ensign Gross whispered.

"I've got the worst pain, and I just can't get comfortable. Is there any chance I could have a heating pad?"

"Oh, we can't put heat on that fresh incision."

"It's not my abdomen," I groaned. "The pain is in my left leg."

"Let's see what the doctor has ordered for you," she responded as she turned to pull my chart. She flipped through several pages of doctors' scribbling. "There's nothing more I can give you until 2 a.m. I'll have to call the duty doctor about the heating pad."

"Don't wake him up for that. I'll just walk a little to see if it will ease up. Thanks anyway."

Efforts to get to sleep were fruitless. Ensign Gross looked concerned as I walked toward the nurses' station again a couple of hours later.

"Are you still in pain, Mrs. Walker?"

"You bet. And I thought 2 o'clock would never come."

"I can give you a couple more aspirins now, and maybe we can do something to take your mind off the pain. I've caught up with my paperwork, and I have a deck of cards. What card games do you know?"

"I know how to play cribbage, rummy, go fish, and honeymoon bridge," I laughed.

"I haven't played honeymoon bridge since college," she grinned.

"Well, you've played more recently than I have. I haven't played since before my honeymoon."

At 6 a.m. Ensign Gross had to stop our card game to prepare her briefing for the oncoming shift. Besides, I had to go to the bathroom. When I sat down in the stall, my catheter fell into the toilet. My first thought was to push the panic call button to call the nurse. It was then that I realized for the first time that the bathrooms were not equipped with emergency call buttons. My only choice was to revert to my ability to whistle through my teeth. After several loud whistles, Ensign Gross sprinted into the bathroom.

"What's going on, Mrs. Walker?"

"My catheter dropped into the toilet, and I need your help."

Ensign Gross almost doubled over with laughter. "Just leave the catheter, and we'll tell the doctor when he makes his rounds this morning. You certainly have made this an interesting midwatch."

Dr. Norris had a concerned look on his face when he entered my room at 7 a.m. during his morning rounds. "I hear you've had a rough night."

I nodded in agreement.

"You realize, of course, it has been less than 48 hours since you had extremely involved surgery, and you need all the rest you can get. I've discontinued the catheter and ordered some pain medicine and a heating pad for your leg. But you really ought to see the orthopedic doctors about it as soon as possible."

Chapter Four

Two days after my release from the hospital, my mother arrived bearing gifts. Mom is a short, plump, talkative woman whose red hair over time has become dulled by silver strands.

After hugs and kisses all around, her first question was "Why are you limping, Honey?"

"I wish I knew, Mom."

As Jack retrieved her luggage in the baggage area, I recounted to her in a long narration the problems with my leg since May.

The two weeks Mom spent with us during my "recuperation" were full of fun, chatter, and shopping.

The night before my mother was scheduled to fly home, Mom, Jack, and I were in the kitchen preparing dinner. As I leaned against the stove to stir the vegetables on the back burner, I made a discovery.

"You know, guys, I don't match anymore!"

"What do you mean?" Jack asked with a confused look.

"My left leg has a lump in it!"

"How can you tell?" Mom asked.

"When I stand next to the stove, my left leg touches before

my right one. And I can actually feel a knot when I rub it. Come over here and see if you can feel it."

Both Mom and Jack agreed that there seemed to be a lump in my left thigh.

"When do you go back to Dr. Jackson?" Jack inquired.

"Next week. And I'm going to tell him I want some action."

Our conversation about my leg was abruptly ended when the kids burst into the room hungry as wolves.

The next day we took Mom to the airport to catch her flight back to Minneapolis. After she said goodbye and began walking down the ramp to her plane, she turned and said: "Don't forget to tell that doctor—we want some action, Jackson!"

Jack and I chuckled as we waved goodbye to her.

The Rheumatology Clinic waiting room was overflowing with patients as I walked in for my appointment and made my way to one of the few remaining seats. After waiting for what seemed like an eternity, Dr. Jackson called my name.

"Sorry you had to wait so long. This seems to be the season for bone problems," he said apologetically.

"All your blood work seems to be normal," he began. "But I notice you're favoring your left leg. Has it gotten worse?"

"Yes, I think it has. I don't know if you remember or not, but I had a hysterectomy last month. I had no trouble recuperating from that. However, I had a severe pain attack in my leg, and the gynecologist gave me some pain medication for it," I recounted as I showed him the medicine bottle. "I've also discovered that I have a lump in my thigh."

"H'mm, let's take a look at it."

After feeling the lump, he sat back in his chair and wrinkled his brow in thought.

"My best educated guess is that it is a knot in your muscle like a charley horse. You must have pulled or strained a muscle at some time. And with constant use, it has taken this long to show up."

"So you think I need to go back to orthopedics?" I inquired.

"No. I don't think that's necessary. Time will take care of it.

One thing I know for sure is that it isn't a rheumatology problem. I'll just treat it symptomatically with a muscle relaxant and another prescription for pain medication. If you continue to have problems, go back to the orthopedic walk-in clinic."

As I drove home, I had a sinking feeling that Dr. Jackson's "treatment" was not going to be a panacea.

The time between mid-October and Thanksgiving passed quickly. Our kids have always loved Halloween, and this year was no exception. They were also anxiously awaiting Thanksgiving since we had invited Judy Husebo, one of their all-time favorite persons, and her fiance, Gale Parks, to share turkey day with us.

I first met Judy in 1953 when my parents moved to Minneapolis from Waterloo, Iowa. It was friendship at first sight, and I literally became an extension of her family.

During spring break of my senior year in high school, Judy's parents invited me to accompany them to Fort Myers, Florida, on their annual Florida vacation. We spent three glorious weeks sunning, swimming, sight-seeing, and burning up the golf links in her parent's golf cart.

Jack jokingly refers to Judy and me as the odd couple. Judy is tall, willowy, quiet, and introspective. Conversely, I am short, small, boisterous, and an extrovert. But somehow our friendship works.

Our Thanksgiving Day equalled all our expectations. Of course, none of us thought we ever wanted to eat again. But when the phone rang the next day with an invitation to join our neighbors for dinner at a new pizza place in Gaithersburg, we couldn't resist. Lou and Hilda Ponder were exceptional neighbors. They treated all of us like family. Hilda was a Maryland native, and Lou described himself as a "Georgia cracker." They had lived in the Washington, D.C. area for many years, and they knew where to go to get the best food, service, or product.

As we waited for our pizza order to arrive, I began to feel the familiar nagging pain in my left leg. I tried to ignore the pain by engaging in conversation with the Ponders, Jack, and the kids. But by the time we left the restaurant, the pain was all consuming.

"Honey, I think we've got to go straight to the emergency room at Bethesda," I said as we got in our car.

"That pain pill you took didn't help?" Jack inquired.

"No. And the pain is real bad. I don't think I'll be able to get through the night without some stronger medication."

Jack dropped me off at the door of the emergency room, and he and the kids circled the driveway to find a parking spot. I explained to the troll on duty my history of visits to see Dr. Jackson. I was told to wait until the on-call orthopedic doctor could be reached. As I turned to take a seat, I noticed Barbara Brown's husband nervously pacing outside one of the emergency room cubicles.

"Hello, Ben. What on earth are you doing here?"

Ben looked at me with red-rimmed eyes. "Barbara's had a massive stroke. She's in critical condition."

About that time Jack arrived, and we both expressed our concern. Our conversation was interrupted by the troll calling my name. He said the orthopedic on-call had approved a stronger pain medication. If that didn't help, he instructed me to return to orthopedic walk-in after the Thanksgiving holidays.

David's birthday is always right around Thanksgiving, usually a day or two after. This year, however, he got an unwanted birthday present—viral pneumonia—which took about two weeks to run its course.

As soon as the pneumonia diagnosis was confirmed, Jack and I became concerned about whether or not my parents' planned trip to visit us for Christmas might be in jeopardy. My father, David Crawford, was a severe asthmatic; therefore, exposure to any respiratory illness had to be avoided at all costs. But we were assured by David's doctor that his pneumonia should be behind him by Christmas. So preparations for a big family Christmas went forward with baking, shopping, and wrapping gifts.

By this time, my left leg had deteriorated to the point where I was in extreme agony most of the time. To make matters worse, my right leg had begun to ache almost as badly as my left.

It was especially painful to get up from a seated position and begin to walk.

One night in early December after putting the kids to bed, Jack helped me down the stairs.

"Mary, darlin', you've got to do something about your limp before your folks come. They're going to be very concerned."

"I know. I walk just like Frankenstein. All I need are a couple of electrodes on my head," I laughed.

"Now don't joke about this, Mary. Promise me you'll do something about it soon."

I fully intended to go back to the doctor, but when Jack came home two days later with chills and a high fever, I decided my return trip would have to wait a while. Our fears were realized a couple of days later when Jack's illness was confirmed as viral pneumonia. We notified my parents, and they reluctantly cancelled their Christmas trip to Maryland.

Jack had a rough couple of weeks with his illness. As is not uncommon for an adult, his pneumonia was much worse than David's. Although he was not hospitalized, he was ordered to stay in bed and to keep his fever down with aspirin.

A couple of days after the kids began their Christmas holidays, we got ready to go shopping for our Christmas tree.

"Mary, I really don't feel like getting out of bed, and you can hardly walk," Jack moaned as he saw the kids in their coats.

"Oh, now don't be a Scrooge. The kids are looking forward to it, and they'll be out of your hair for a couple of hours. It'll be lots of fun."

"Can't I talk you out of it this year?" he pleaded.

"No, we've always had a real tree, and the kids and I would be disappointed if we didn't have one this year."

The kids and I began singing "Frostie the Snowman" as we piled into the car.

As we approached our fourth Christmas tree lot, it had begun to snow. I told the kids we had to find our tree here and get home because Dad would be worried about us.

After stumping around the lot and holding up dozens of trees for inspection, I pulled one from the pile and held it up for the kid's approval. They assured me that at last we had found the "perfect" tree.

We lugged the tree to the car, and after stuffing it in the trunk, two feet of pine still stuck out. By now the snow was falling heavier. As I tried to back out, my heart sank as I realized we were stuck. The tires whined as they spun in place, sinking deeper into the snow. I knew the only way out would be to try to rock back and forth. In desperation, I opened the door and stuck out my sore left leg to help push out. Miraculously, after several minutes, we rocked free. With "Jingle Bells" ringing in my ears, we headed for home.

As soon as I unlocked the door, the kids burst into the house. "Daddy! Daddy! We've got the best Christmas tree in the world! Come look at it!"

Jack got out of bed and walked to the top of the stairs, looking down at us. "I sure am glad to see you," he said. "I was beginning to worry."

"Jack, honey, do you feel like getting the tree out of the car and mounting it for us?" I asked.

"Sure. I took a couple of aspirins about an hour ago, and my fever has gone down."

Jack dressed in his warmest clothes and braved the outdoors for the first time in over a week. As he carried the tree from the car to the garage, I thought smugly what a great choice we had made since it looked so full and beautiful.

Jack began struggling to get the tree in the Christmas tree stand. Every time he tried to get it to stand alone, it would topple over.

Exhausted after several attempts, Jack looked at me in frustration. "This tree will never stand up. It's lop-sided. Look, the whole trunk is crooked."

"Well, what are we gonna do?" I cried.

"We have two choices—sink it in concrete or cut it up for firewood."

"Oh, no! There's gotta be something else we can do."

Jack thought for a moment. "We could anchor it in a bucket filled with rocks. But I don't feel like going rock hunting right now. I've got to get back to bed. I'm aching all over. Maybe I'll feel like doing it tomorrow."

"Okay," I agreed. "Let's go in the house. You go back to bed, and I'll start dinner."

As soon as Jack got settled in bed, armed with a ten-gallon, galvanized bucket from the garage, I headed for a new house under construction at the end of our block.

Several days later Jack and I were having coffee after dinner in front of our newly-decorated tree. Except for the rather large base, surprisingly it looked almost normal.

The pain in my legs for the past week had been almost unbearable. But with Christmas approaching, I tried to put it out of my mind. As I took the coffee cups back to the kitchen, Jack observed my steadily deteriorating walk.

"Mary, darlin', your legs look like they're really bothering you tonight."

Unable to mask the torture any longer, I turned to Jack in tears.

"I don't think I can stand it anymore. I'm in constant pain 24 hours a day."

"For heaven's sake, you've got to get some relief," Jack said as he attempted to comfort me.

"Tomorrow you're going into that hospital, and you're going to keep going in every day until we get to the bottom of this."

With Jack feeling better and able to look after the kids in my absence, I started out bright and early the next morning to try to solve the mystery of my aching legs.

Much to my surprise, I discovered that Dr. Allen was still the orthopedic walk-in physician. As he called my name, I struggled to get to my feet and to walk toward his office.

As I sat down, I began: "I'm sorry to be such a thorn in your side. But I'm getting progressively worse. I just have to find out what's wrong with me."

"Oh, I remember you now. I thought we had your problem

solved. What did they find out in rheumatology?"

"Dr. Jackson said it wasn't a rheumatology problem, and he's been treating it symptomatically. He said to come back to orthopedics if I weren't getting better."

Dr. Allen flipped through my medical record in silence for a few minutes. Finally, he looked up. "Let's get some fresh X-rays and see what's going on."

After a two-hour wait for X-rays, I stumped back to Dr. Allen's clinic.

"I don't see any problem from the X-rays," he began. "The best I can do is to adjust your medication. If that doesn't help, come back."

Each morning for the next four days I showed up at Dr. Allen's clinic trying to get some relief. Even the stronger pain medications he had prescribed were ineffective.

Finally, on the Friday before Christmas as I walked into the clinic, Dr. Allen spotted me and ushered me directly into office.

"Mrs. Walker," Dr. Allen exclaimed in exasperation, "you have been in here every day this week!"

"Well, you know the old saying: 'the squeaky wheel gets the grease.'"

"There really is nothing more we can do for you. We've X-rayed you from head to toe, and I've come to the conclusion that your problem is not physical. I think your problem is mental."

I sat in stunned silence as he continued.

"I'm referring you to the psychiatric clinic."

Chapter Five

"The Eyes of Texas are upon you, all the live long day. . ." sang out the fans in Dallas in unison with the Longhorn Band. The 1974 New Year's Day Cotton Bowl classic between Texas and Nebraska was getting underway as Jack and I settled down in front of the TV. Since The University of Texas is Jack's alma mater, we are ardent fans of all sporting events involving the Longhorns.

By half time, with the game not going too well for the 'Horns, I decided to take our beagle, Snoopy, for a walk in the woods near our house.

Snoopy had been a surprise birthday present to Jack from the kids and me. While he was on a business trip to California, we decided it was entirely too lonely without a pet. So even though Jack was not particularly fond of dogs at that point, we rationalized that getting a dog would be our reward for having to stay home. And, besides, Jack would learn to love a dog in time.

In the year and a half that we had owned Snoopy, a routine developed in which she was walked several times a week. On these outings, I was usually accompanied by David and Amy, along with their best neighborhood friends, Kevin and Brian Sullivan, and their dog, Daisy.

Since this day was cold, damp, and windy, only David and Brian chose to venture out with the dogs and me. When we got to the wood's edge, I unleashed Snoopy, and the boys and dogs charged ahead, unencumbered by my slower pace.

After about 20 minutes of romping in the woods, I was chilled to the bone. I yelled to the boys to leash the dogs so we could start heading for home. At that moment, Snoopy caught a scent and took off running back into the woods with David in hot pursuit. Brian and I turned and started heading back in the direction of home. As we started down a small hill, my feet slipped on the wet grass, and I fell head over heels like a rag doll, finally coming to rest at the bottom.

"Are you okay, Mrs. Walker?" Brian inquired, barely able to conceal his amusement over my apparent clumsiness.

"Oh, Brian," I moaned, "I think I'm going to need some help. Will you please go back to the house to get Mr. Walker?"

He and Daisy raced off in a flash.

As I lay on the ground looking up at the gray sky, I thought to myself, "I've really done it this time. I must have severely damaged something, and I'll probably be out of whack for a couple of weeks."

After what seemed like an endless wait, I heard Jack calling my name.

"I'm over here at the bottom of this little hill, Honey."

As he came nearer, I could see from his expression that he wasn't happy with the situation.

"How's the game going?" I inquired, trying to divert his attention from my awkward predicament.

"Not well. But I'm not concerned about that right now."

"Did David and Snoopy get home okay?"

"Yes, but you wouldn't have been in this situation if it weren't for that damn dog. Let's see if we can get you on your feet."

After a painful struggle, Jack got me into a standing position.

"Put your arm on my shoulder, and hop on your good leg,"

Jack instructed as he held me steady around my waist.

"I don't have a good leg," I tearfully replied. "I can't hop anywhere."

"What in the world have you done?"

"I don't know. I'm in terrible pain. I must have pulled something badly."

"Then I'll just carry you home."

"Oh, no! You'll hurt your back. Isn't there some other way to get back?"

Jack lowered me to a sitting position on the ground and thought for a moment. "How about me going to get the kids' little red wagon? Do you think you could stand riding in that?"

"Oh, that's a great idea."

"I'll be back as soon as possible," he yelled as he jogged off in the direction of home.

After a few minutes I was delighted to hear the rumbling of the wagon over the rough ground.

"Here's your chariot, me Lady," Jack laughed as he crested the hill, pulling my rescue vehicle behind him.

Jack gently lifted me into the wagon. "Hang on. I'll try to make this as smooth as possible."

As we began this strange journey, my teeth were clinched and my knuckles were white from my firm grasp on the wagon's sides.

After bumping along for about 50 feet, I yelled "Hojotoho!"

"You sound like Brünnhilde. What's wrong?" Jack asked as he stopped the wagon.

"I feel like one of the Valkyries on her horse. Is there any chance we could take the bumps slower?"

After several more minutes, much to my relief, we arrived at our house. Jack opened the front door and carried me to the steps leading to the upstairs bedrooms.

"Let me round up the kids, and we'll be on our way to the hospital as soon as we can," Jack said breathlessly.

"No, Honey. If I could just make it upstairs and soak in a hot tub, I know I'll feel a lot better. I'm sure it's just a bad pull," I said confidently as I scooted on my fanny to the next higher step. By the time I got to the top of the stairs, Jack had filled the tub half full of hot water. As he helped lower me into the soothing warmth, I felt sure this treatment would be the solution to my problem.

After about 20 minutes, Jack popped his head back into the steamy room. "Are you feeling any better?"

"Yeah, I think so. Maybe I'd better get out now. I feel like I'm turning into a raisin."

As I moved to position myself to get out of the tub, I felt like *rigor mortis* had set in. I knew there was no way either Jack or I would be able to get me out.

"Here, let me lift you," Jack offered as he bent his body over me.

"That's impossible. I'm just dead weight. You'll break your back. We've got to get some help."

"Who in the world can we get with you naked in the tub?"

"Don't you think Dick Sullivan would come over to help? I'll dress down as far as possible. And then I'll cover up 'possible' before he comes."

Jack reluctantly agreed with my suggestion since our options were limited. Shortly after Jack's telephone call, Dick was ringing the doorbell.

Dick Sullivan was a tall, thin, dark-haired man with a pensive countenance which complimented his quiet personality.

After assessing the situation, Jack and Dick decided to make an "Indian chair" with their arms and hands and to lift me from the tub to our bed. After Jack helped me get dressed, they utilized their improvised seat again to carry me downstairs and out to our car.

As Jack started the car, Dick volunteered that he and his wife, Sheila, would watch David and Amy while we were at the hospital.

The emergency room at Bethesda Naval Hospital normally moves at a frantic pace. However, at 6 p.m. on New Year's Day, it was more like a morgue. Jack was able to commandeer a wheelchair and a corpsman to help get me out of the car.

After hearing the story of my fall and taking my vital signs, the emergency room doctor sent us to X-ray.

Jack and the technician on duty lifted me onto the cold, hard X-ray table. Trying to get my body into a flat position after being drawn up in pain for several hours was a herculean task. After having several agonizing views taken, I was shoehorned into the wheelchair once again and told to wait for the radiologist's report.

"How are you holding up, Mary, darlin'?" Jack inquired.

"Okay, I guess. I'm still hanging in there," I smiled weakly as we positioned ourselves so that we could see into the X-ray reviewing room.

The radiologist on duty was closely examining my X-ray pictures on his lighted review panel. He rotated the half dozen films several times, viewing them in different sequences. Finally, he gathered up the X-rays and emerged from the room and approached us with a puzzled look on his face.

"How old are you, Mrs. Walker?"

"Thirty-seven," I replied without hesitation.

"There's something very unusual about your X-rays. You have the bones of an 80-year-old woman. Have you had a hysterectomy?"

"Yes, last September."

"Are you on hormones?"

"Yes."

"Well, your bones look like you have osteoporosis."

"What's that?" Jack and I asked simultaneously.

"That's where your bones have a porous, thinned appearance. It's very common in older women."

"Is that what's causing my problem?" I asked anxiously.

"It may be a contributing factor. But your biggest problem right now is a fractured right hip."

Jack and I were still in a daze as we returned to the emergency room with the radiologist's report. In my wildest dreams I couldn't imagine a 37-year-old woman breaking her hip. I always thought that affliction was the sole province of the geriatric set.

After reviewing the report, the emergency room doctor directed us to admissions and then to the orthopedic ward where the duty orthopedic doctor would be waiting for us.

Moments after our arrival in my hospital room, a muscular, good-looking man about my age came in.

"Mrs. Walker? I'm Dr. Ryan."

"Hi, Dr. Ryan. I bet we tore you away from the football game."

"That's okay," he grinned. "My team isn't winning anyway."

"Neither did ours," Jack piped in.

"I've just been flipping through your medical record, and I see you've graced the walk-in clinic quite a few times."

"Yeah. I've beat a pretty hot path between our house and the clinic during the past six months."

Our conversation was interrupted by the orthopedic technician arriving loaded down with weights and pulleys.

"I'm going to put you in traction and give you some pain medication to make you more comfortable," Dr. Ryan continued. "We'll schedule surgery to repair your hip for the day after tomorrow."

After Dr. Ryan left, Jack made a list of the personal necessities I wanted him to bring for my hospital stay. By now the jungle gym in the form of traction gear was in place, and I was feeling some relief from the pain. Jack kissed me goodnight and hurried off to retrieve our kids from the Sullivans.

Chapter Six

The hospital corridors were still dark as I was being pushed toward the operating room on a gurney. I wondered if anyone else in Washington, D.C. could be up at this early hour other than surgeons and milkmen. As the doors of the operating suite swung open, a frigid blast of air hit me head on.

"Brr! This is too much like Minnesota. You don't have a spare blanket, do you?" I asked through my chattering teeth as the attendant parked my gurney.

"No, but I've got a hot sheet," the corpsman responded as he spread the warmth over me.

As I was being transferred to the operating table, the green-masked staff members were busy with their final preparations. My last recollection of the OR was when the anesthesiologist put a mask over my mouth and nose and instructed me to take ten deep breaths.

Although I was awake from time to time in the recovery room, I wasn't fully conscious until I was wheeled back to my room about mid-afternoon. Jack's smiling face was there to greet me. He held me tightly for several seconds and kissed me gently on the neck.

"I'm so glad it's over. I love you, Sweetheart," he whispered.

"I love you too. I don't know what I'd do without you," I responded.

"How do you feel?"

"Pretty good. I don't think I could run the hundred yard dash right now. But I'll be fine in a few days."

Jack brought me up to date on David and Amy and explained that Sheila Sullivan would meet them after school. He also told me about calling my folks.

A knock at the door interrupted our discussion. It was Dr. Ryan, accompanied by a distinguished-looking man around 50. He had steely-blue, but compassionate, eyes and salt and pepper hair. Dr. Ryan introduced his companion as Dr. Slimmons, Chief of Orthopedics.

"How're you feeling, Mrs. Walker?" Dr. Ryan inquired.

"Please call me Mary. I'm doing okay. How did the surgery go?"

"Technically your surgery went fine. We put three pins in your hip." Dr. Ryan seemed lost for words as he looked out the window.

"However, we found some abnormal-looking cells," Dr. Slimmons interjected.

"Abnormal cells? What do you mean by that?" Jack inquired.

"The bone and tissue we sent to pathology didn't look normal. We'll have to wait for the pathological report to determine if there's a problem."

"I wish we could have brought you more definitive news. But we'll keep our fingers crossed and hope for the best," Dr. Ryan concluded as the surgeons left the room.

Jack and I sat in silence, trying to guess what might be wrong. Our solitude was broken when Mrs. Webster, my roommate, was wheeled back into the room after having had hip surgery. She had checked in late the night before. She was a tall, gray-haired lady in her late sixties. She was babbling incoherently as Jack kissed me goodnight and left to pick up the kids.

The Fat Lady Hasn't Sung

The combination of anesthesia and pain medication helped me get to sleep rather quickly in spite of the unsettling news.

At 2 a.m. I was suddenly awakened by Mrs. Webster's loud cries for help.

"Help! We've got to get out of here! The horses are stampeding around the room! I'll come and get you, Mary."

"No, Mrs. Webster! Just stay in bed." I urged her as I frantically searched for the call button.

Within seconds a corpsman arrived and attempted to calm Mrs. Webster down. She continued to hallucinate: "Tie that horse down! Look out! Don't let him step on you!"

The corpsman trotted out of the room looking for reinforcements. A few minutes later he returned with the night nurse and another corpsman. While the nurse injected Mrs. Webster with a sedative, the two corpsmen put her in restraints.

Mrs. Webster's hallucinations continued through the next day. By the time Jack arrived, her earlier sedations had begun to wear off.

Jack's mood was surprisingly upbeat as he greeted me with a long kiss. He told me about the kids' doings and about his telephone conversation with his parents. I told him about my roommate's equestrian experiences the night before. Our visit was abruptly interrupted by Mrs. Webster.

"Be careful! There's a huge spider on the wall over your bed! Lookout! It's going to get you! Help!"

Jack quickly excused himself and disappeared out the door. After a few minutes he returned, followed shortly by the head nurse, Mrs. Collins. She was a fine-figured woman of about 45 years with flaming red hair.

"Mrs. Walker, we're going to round you up and head you down the hall to another room where I think you'll be more comfortable," Mrs. Collins grinned with obvious tongue in cheek.

A few minutes later I was settled in my new room. For now, I was the only occupant.

"Nice, quiet room isn't it?" Jack asked.

"Yeah. Gee, I wonder why they moved me?"

Jack smiled roguishly as he kissed me goodnight. "I guess we'll never know."

During morning rounds the next day, Dr. Ryan informed me that Dr. Perlin, Chief of Oncology, would be coming by to see me mid-afternoon to discuss the pathological report. He said he would call Jack so he could be there with me.

Jack left work early and arrived in my room just before 2 p.m. We were both optimistically apprehensive about the pathological report. Perhaps the abnormal-looking cells were benign. Or maybe the orthopedic doctors had been unduly cautious.

Our speculation was suspended by the sound of a light knock at the door. A short, slightly-built man in his early forties wearing rimless glasses was standing at the door. The horseshoe fringe of his traditional male-pattern baldness had started to turn gray. His demeanor was one of seriousness.

"Commander and Mrs. Walker? I'm Dr. Perlin from oncology. I'm here to decipher and discuss your pathological report."

"Before we begin, could you tell us what oncology is?" Jack queried.

"Oncology is that branch of medicine which specializes in the treatment of cancer," Dr. Perlin explained. "I'm here to let you know that the pathological report came back positive."

"Does that mean that I have cancer?" I inquired in a quavering voice.

"Yes, I'm afraid it does."

"What kind of cancer is it? Can it be treated?" Jack implored in rapid succession.

Dr. Perlin responded with a long medical term. The only part either Jack or I recognized was the word "carcinoma."

By the time he uttered the word "carcinoma," the sound seemed as though it was being transmitted from a long distance, as if it were coming from the bottom of a well. Then, all the voices, including my own, began to sound like echoes around me.

"Dr. Perlin, what type of treatment do you plan for this kind of cancer?" I choked out in spite of the lump in my throat.

"Unfortunately, this cancer does not respond well to any type of treatment." Dr. Perlin was now becoming quite uncomfortable. "But we're going to fight it with everything we've got available to us. You know, we're making great strides every day in cancer treatment."

"Is there any way you can predict how long I might have to live?"

"Of course there are always exceptions," Dr. Perlin responded. "However, for patients with this type of cancer, the average longevity is about six months."

I felt like I had just been hit by a sledgehammer or stabbed in my heart. The pins were completely knocked out from under me. All I wanted was for Dr. Perlin to leave so I could cry.

Jack asked Dr. Perlin a few more questions and thanked him for coming by. Their conversation seemed to be coming from a long distance away. It was almost as if I were having an out-of-body experience. I felt as if I were in a trance.

It seemed like several minutes had elapsed before I felt Jack embrace me. As soon as I felt his warm strength holding me, I burst into tears: "I don't want to die! I have so much to live for."

"I know, Sweetheart. I know."

He held me for several minutes patting me on the back as tears racked both our bodies.

"Who's going to take care of the kids? They're so young. How are they ever going to understand?" I wept.

After a long silence, I felt Jack's sobs subsiding. It seemed like several more minutes passed before one of us spoke again.

"How could this be happening to me? I've taken such good care of myself. What have I done to deserve this?" I asked as Jack embraced me.

"You haven't done anything, Honey. We're just going to have to fight it. We've known several people who've beaten cancer." Jack said in an assuring voice.

"I can't bear to think of David and Amy without a mother," I sobbed again.

"Mary, darlin', we've got to get hold of ourselves. We're going to fight this. And you're going to be the exception!"

"I'll try. I'll try my best."

"Dr. Perlin said that he couldn't start treatments until they find the primary source of the cancer. He feels the cancer started in some internal organ and has spread to your hip," Jack explained.

"Is that what he said just before he left the room?"

"Yeah. And he and Dr. Slimmons are ordering a battery of tests to begin as soon as possible, probably tomorrow or the day after."

By the time Jack was ready to leave, I had pretty much regained my composure. Realizing this, Jack broached a subject which apparently was weighing heavily on him.

"What am I going to tell your parents?"

"I don't want to tell them about the cancer yet. Let's wait until they find the primary source."

"Why don't I give them your phone number here so they can talk to you direct?" Jack proposed, sounding relieved.

To be honest, that was the first time I realized I had a phone in my room.

True to Dr. Perlin's prediction, the tests began the next day. About 10 a.m. a corpsman pushing a gurney showed up to transport me to the gynecology ward. (Since I wasn't able to walk, all of my subsequent excursions around the hospital were made by gurney).

When I entered the GYN area, I heard a familiar voice: "I'm happy to see you're still smiling, Mrs. Walker."

"Hi, Dr. Norris. I think we're finally getting to the bottom of my leg pain."

"That's good," Dr. Norris replied. "Since you've just had your hip fixed, I'll be very careful."

After a brief examination, Dr. Norris stated that everything looked okay. He said he didn't think there was a gynecological source of the cancer. But just to be on the safe side, he indicated he would review all the tissue slides from my hysterectomy and then send a complete report to orthopedics.

For the next two weeks, every morning and afternoon, some

part of my body was being examined by hand, film, scope, needle, tube, or scan.

There was the inevitable upper and lower gastrointestinal series. But perhaps the two most uncomfortable tests were the proctoscope and endoscope exams, the latter of which must be what swallowing a garden hose would be like. Closely rivaling those two tests in discomfort was a bone marrow aspiration in which a long needle is pushed through the skin, tissue, and bone into the pelvis to withdraw marrow.

Most of the other tests were more fascinating than uncomfortable. The arteriogram and the brain, kidney, liver, and thyroid scans all revealed the workings of parts of my body which heretofore had been locked up by the secrecy of nature.

Each day during Jack's visit I briefed him on the procedures involved in the latest test. While we were speculating that I might run out of body parts if these tests continued much longer, Dr. Slimmons entered my room on his afternoon rounds.

"We think we may have found the primary source," he began.

"Good! Where is it?" I asked.

"Well, as you know, all of your tests have come back normal. Except for one. Your thyroid scan shows a hot spot or possible tumor."

Dr. Slimmons pulled an X-ray out of an envelope under his arm, shoved it into a lighted screen on my wall, and stared intently at the black and white shadows for several seconds, puffing on his ever-present pipe.

"Our latest X-rays reveal a fracture in your left hip, as well as the break we found earlier on your right side," he said as he pointed to an almost invisible hairline mark on the bone. "You probably broke it during your fall. But we didn't notice it until now."

"Do you suppose that weakness in the bone could have caused all my pain for the past eight months?" I asked with a slight sense of relief.

"Possibly," Dr. Slimmons speculated thoughtfully, still drawing deeply on his pipe. "We have scheduled the thyroid surgery for the day after tomorrow. Since that's a fairly short procedure, we would like your permission to fix your hip at the same time, while you're already under anesthesia."

I looked at Jack, and he shrugged his shoulders: "Why not?"

"Okay, Dr. Slimmons. It looks like I'm going to get two for the price of one!"

Chapter Seven

As the anesthesia started to wear off, my eyes began to focus on the people and objects in the recovery room. Two green-clothed attendants busied themselves over me, taking my blood pressure and adjusting the humidifier delivering mist to my throat area.

As I looked around the room, another patient, a man on my right, also appeared to be coming around from his anesthesia. The bed to my left was empty. A television set was hanging on the wall nearby with its sound muted and a basketball game in progress. After several minutes the network took a commercial break. I immediately recognized the commercial as the popular Schlitz Malt Liquor ad depicting a large bull crashing through a wall.

"Look out! Run! Here he comes again!" the man on my right screamed wildly as he struggled to free himself from his medical entanglements. The recovery room staff rushed to restrain him just as he managed to get his right leg over the side of the bed. It was then that I noticed his left leg had been amputated just above the knee.

"It's okay, Mark," one of the corpsmen reassured him as he retaped his i.v. "It's just a commercial."

"I thought it was happening all over again," Mark continued to sob hysterically.

"You're safe here. You're not in Spain anymore," the corpsmen reassured him.

After several minutes, Mark calmed down and apparently drifted off to sleep.

The corpsman turned and leaned over my bed. "Everything all right here, Mrs. Walker?"

"What's the matter?" I croaked, realizing for the first time how sore my throat was.

"Mark is stationed at Rota, Spain. He was gored during the running of the bulls through the streets of Pamplona. I guess in his groggy state he relived the accident through the TV commercial."

I thought to myself what a terrible price to pay for getting up close and personal with a bull.

As the recovery room returned to normal, I drifted in and out of sleep for the next couple of hours.

"Are you awake, Mary?" a familiar voice inquired. Dr. Slimmons, still in scrubs, was patting my hand.

"How did my 'two-fer' go?" I smiled.

"Well, I've got some good news and some bad news. Which would you like first?"

"I could stand some good news about now."

"The good news is the spot on your thyroid turned out to be a benign tumor."

"Oh, that *is* good news!" I squawked.

"Now the bad news. We found a massive malignant tumor from the knee to the pelvis," Dr. Slimmons began hesitantly. "That obviously is the primary source we've been looking for," he continued, fidgeting with his surgical mask. "We removed as much of the tumor as possible and sent a big slice to pathology. It looked like raw fish."

"Is that how you could tell it was malignant?"

"Yeah. It had that characteristic look of cancerous tissue." By this time he was visibly more uneasy with this conversation. "We also ran into another problem. Your bone was so soft and porous that we could push the nails right through it. It was just like Swiss cheese. Therefore, it was inoperable, and we couldn't repair the fracture."

"I know this sounds strange," I began, choosing my words carefully. "But I actually feel vindicated."

"What do you mean?" Dr. Slimmons obviously was puzzled by my remark.

"The pain in my left leg was legitimate after all, even though Dr. Allen believed it was psychosomatic. I can't understand why no one saw the tumor on X-rays."

Dr. Slimmons maintained his poker face. "Tumors don't show up on X-rays, Mary. You have to use scanning machines. Even then, we miss some. Oh, by the way, the general surgeon who did your thyroid will drop by to see you on the ward in a couple of days."

Dr. Slimmons turned to go. "I'm sure you'd like to know that Jack's outside waiting to see you. I'll send him in for a few minutes. I've already briefed him on your surgery, so you won't have to talk so much with your sore throat."

The rest of my time in recovery was uneventful, and I was back in my room before dinner. Much to my surprise, I discovered that I had acquired a roommate during my absence.

Mrs. Spruce was a spherically-shaped woman in her late sixties. Her left leg was missing below the knee. Her eyes seemed to be staring past me as we exchanged introductions. As I was to learn later, she suffered from runaway diabetes which already had claimed her eyesight and one leg. She had been admitted for evaluation and possible amputation of her right leg.

A couple of days after my surgery, during morning rounds, Dr. Slimmons introduced Dr. Gregory, the general surgeon. He was a thin man in his middle thirties with sparse blond hair. His pale countenance made one wonder if he ever got out of the operating room.

After Dr. Slimmons and his orthopedic entourage moved on, Dr. Gregory took charge. "Let's have a look at that incision," he began, as he removed the bandage from my neck. "What a beautiful job!" he exclaimed as he examined the red track across my throat. "Would you like to see it?" he asked as he produced a mirror from the pocket of his white coat.

"It looks to me like I've had a run-in with Jack the Ripper," I countered as I saw the reflection of the angry scar.

"Oh, no! I want to show this to the plastic surgeons," he replied confidently.

About mid-afternoon that day, Dr. Slimmons arrived unexpectedly, accompanied by a familiar face.

"I'm sure you remember Mrs. Walker, don't you Dr. Allen?" Dr. Allen nodded sheepishly. Dr. Slimmons began placing X-rays on the lighted wall panel. After he had flipped up a half dozen pictures, he stepped back, his gaze transfixed, and drew heavily on his pipe.

"This first X-ray was taken in May and the last one in December," Dr. Slimmons began, speaking directly to Dr. Allen. "With these X-rays all in a row, do you notice any bone change?"

Dr. Allen stared intently at each picture. By the time he came to the last X-ray, he lowered his face, pale with embarrassment. "Yes, Sir. There is a difference between the first and the most recent. But the change is so subtle you wouldn't notice it in just one view."

"I agree," Dr Slimmons nodded in assent. "But if you had taken the time to compare each new set of X-rays with her earlier ones, we probably would have been able to diagnose her problem much earlier," he continued. By now his voice had become quite forceful. "That's why we maintain X-ray files."

Dr. Allen looked out the window across the hospital grounds as Dr. Slimmons wound up his admonition. After a long pause, he lifted his downcast eyes and turned to face me. "I'm terribly sorry, Mrs. Walker. I know I can't make it up to you now." His words became more difficult. "But at least I've learned something from your ordeal. It'll never happen again to any other patient of mine."

I smiled trying to reassure the two doctors that I wasn't bitter. "I'm just glad that everyone now knows that my pain wasn't all in my head."

As Dr. Slimmons turned to leave, he said the new pathological report would be back tomorrow.

The next day Jack arrived at his usual time anxious to hear my medical update and full of news about the latest happenings at home.

When he arrived home yesterday, Amy met him with a bloody lip, and David was bombarding two neighbor kids with rocks. As he tried to get David to cease fire, he noticed the neighbor kids had adult reinforcements in the form of their live-in maid, Patranilla. When Jack saw Patranilla hurling rocks at our kids, his "frontier mentality" came to the fore. (I have teased Jack all of our married life about his trait of changing from being an easy-going individual most of the time to a firebrand when he perceives someone is threatening his family or his space. Like most Texans, you can only push him so far, and then he digs in his boots.)

"What did you do to stop it?" I asked in disbelief.

"Well, my Spanish is pretty rusty, but I managed to remember enough, especially cuss-words, to let Patranilla know I wasn't happy."

"What did you say?"

" '*No tire piedras a los niños,*' plus some expletives I learned as a kid in San Antonio."

"Well, what does that mean?"

"Don't throw rocks at the children."

"What was her reaction?"

"When I spoke in the vernacular, she knew I meant business and beat a hasty retreat."

"Were the kids hurt?"

"No, not from the rocks. Amy got her bloody lip from falling trying to avoid getting hit. But she's okay."

It was amazing to me how Jack was bearing up under the pressure. Not only did he visit me each day (sometimes for several hours at a time), but he performed his job, looked after two small children, and managed a home, all at the same time. In addition, he spent his lunch break waiting in line to buy gasoline.

"Oh, good, you're both here," Dr. Perlin began as he entered the room with an uncharacteristically broad smile. I've got some wonderful news for you."

"I don't have cancer?" I asked hopefully.

"Well, yes you do," he continued to smile. "But the good news is that you have an entirely different type of cancer than we first thought."

"Why is that good news?" Jack asked, eager for something hopeful.

"The larger sample of the tumor from your last surgery proved conclusively that you have a lymphoma type cancer instead of a carcinoma."

"Doesn't that involve the lymph glands?" I asked, still slightly skeptical.

"Normally it does. But you have a rare form of that type of cancer called hystiocytic lymphoma. And, in your case, it's even more unusual because it apparently attacks just the bone."

"I still don't see why that's good news," Jack persisted.

"Because lymphomas respond well to radiation therapy, and we're making good progress on it using chemotherapy treatments," Dr. Perlin responded almost euphorically.

"Does this improve my survival chances?"

"It certainly does! Generally, most lymphoma patients have about a 30 percent chance of surviving five years. However, in individual cases, no one knows for sure."

By now the good news was beginning to soak in.

"When can I start the treatments?" I asked anxiously.

"We plan to start radiation treatments as soon as your incision has healed enough, probably in about two weeks."

When Dr. Perlin left, Jack held me tightly, his feeling of relief obvious.

After several minutes he loosened his embrace, kissed me gently, and looked at me through misty eyes.

The Fat Lady Hasn't Sung

I smiled happily and whispered, "Honey, I believe my death sentence may be commuted to life."

Chapter Eight

"We'll continue with part two of *As the World Turns* in just a moment," the announcer intoned from the television set.

Although Mrs. Spruce was legally blind, she enjoyed listening to the soap operas. A daily routine had developed in which I described to her what each of the characters was doing as he or she spoke. I had become very adept at watching television for two people.

Suddenly a loud clanging sound pierced the normal din of the hall.

"Oh! Mary! What's happening?" Mrs. Spruce asked in a trembling voice.

"I'm not really sure. It might be a fire alarm."

The hall suddenly became alive with people scurrying past our door. I saw numerous patients—some on crutches, others in casts, and a few in wheelchairs—rushing by. Several members of the nursing staff followed in hot pursuit.

By now Mrs. Spruce was in a state of near panic. "I'm calling for help," she shouted as she pushed her button frantically. The parade of patients and staff continued past our door. "No one's answering the call. What can we do?" Mrs. Spruce cried, as the clanging continued.

"There's not much we can do. You can't see or walk. And they won't even let me out of bed with both my hips broken. Guess we'll just have to wait, and hope it's only a drill."

Several minutes later Mrs. Collins whisked into the room. "What do you need?" she asked in response to our call button.

"A little information would be helpful," I chided. "What's all the confusion about?"

"Oh, it's just a fire drill."

"Why didn't someone come for us?"

Mrs. Collins laughed. "Rest assured, if it had been a real fire, you and Mrs. Spruce would have been the first ones off the floor."

"That's a comforting thought. A few minutes ago we thought we'd been left to fry."

"Speaking of frying," she chuckled, "here are your menus for the next three days."

She placed both menus on my table as she left since I always filled out Mrs. Spruce's.

As I checked off our choices, I noticed Cornish game hen was an entree for Sunday. I smiled nostalgically remembering my first encounter with that bird.

In June of 1958 my mother and I flew to Hawaii to visit my sister, Jean, her husband, Bob Gleason, and their new baby, Melinda. My trip was a college graduation gift from my parents one year early. It was my mother's first flight, and the nine-hour leg from Seattle to Honolulu was white-knuckle time for her. Shortly after take-off, the flight attendant instructed us on ditching procedures over water. Female passengers were told to remove their high heels in such an emergency, and any passenger wearing dentures or eyeglasses would have to remove them. After that announcement, my mother was constantly worried about how she would look without teeth, glasses, and shoes. I tried to reassure her that no one would care how she looked if we had to crash in the ocean.

We arrived safely at Honolulu, and we were presented with

the traditional lei by an olive-skinned hula girl in a grass skirt. Little did I realize as I stepped off that plane that I was about to embark on a vacation which would change my life forever.

Jean and Bob had made arrangements with some of their bachelor friends to provide some social life for me during my stay. One of those friends was Dow Berggren, who had attended the same college with them. He had invited us to a dinner dance at Makalapa Commissioned Officers' Mess on my first weekend. When we arrived at the club, Dow informed us that he had asked one of his bachelor friends and his date to join us. As we approached our table, a handsome young man, seated next to an attractive blonde, stood up. He was somewhat taller than medium height and had a muscular, athletic build. Physically, he immediately reminded me of Yul Brynner as he portrayed the king in *The King and I*.

"Hi, I'm Jack Walker," he said, flashing a great smile. His bluish-green eyes were fixed intently on mine.

"Sorry we're a little late," Jean explained, as we took our seats. "My Mom's a little rusty at babysitting."

By chance, I was seated directly across the table from Jack. The conversation ranged from college experiences to travel to military life. I was instantly attracted to this urbane, soft-spoken Texan. I sensed immediately that he was an intense person of considerable intellectual depth. Although I was somewhat embarrassed by his lack of attention to his date, I was pleased that he apparently found me interesting enough to devote most of his conversation to me. I was completely charmed by his breadth of knowledge and his subtle humor. In my mind, I was comparing him to the other guys I had dated and known in college. Unfortunately for them, there was no comparison.

When dinner arrived, I was the first to be served. When the waiter removed the cover from the plate, I glanced down at the food and exclaimed: "Oh, look! The little chicken has socks on."

My companions around the table erupted with laughter. Jean, in an attempt to spare me further embarrassment, told me that our entree was Cornish game hen. And the "socks" were paper decorations attached to the ends of the drumsticks.

After dinner, the orchestra started to play, beginning with a medley of tunes from the musical *South Pacific*. Jack asked me if I'd like to dance. Just as we reached the plumaria-scented dance floor, the song, "Some Enchanted Evening," was starting. As his muscular arm slipped around my waist, we began to glide across the floor. I felt like I was in Heaven!

I looked up at the bright stars from the open-air dance floor. Minnesota, I thought, was never like this. After a brief silence, I broached the subject which had been bothering me: "I hope you didn't think I was a complete hayseed with the Cornish game hen."

Jack began laughing again. "On the contrary, I thought your comment was funny. You are the most unique girl I've ever met."

"I'm glad you think so. I thought I'd made a fool of myself."

"Not at all," Jack continued. "You know, every girl I've dated for the past four years seems to have a world-weary attitude. You are such a refreshing change."

For the next couple of weeks I saw Jack at several other social functions, but he never asked me for a date. I found out later that he had been led to believe that I was attached to a guy at Mankato State. And, furthermore, he didn't want to undercut Dow who, at my sister's behest, was still squiring me around.

Finally, I guess Jack decided to risk his friendship with Dow, and he thought "to heck" with the boy back home. He asked me to go surfing with him at Waikiki Beach.

We arrived at the beach around noon the next day. Jack stripped down to his baby blue, form-fitting boxer swim trunks, revealing a deeply tanned body. My initial impressions about his muscular body were confirmed immediately. In today's vernacular, he was a "hunk!"

Jack and I mounted separate surf boards and began heading out toward the reef where we could see the larger waves breaking. Once out in the deeper water, we turned our boards toward shore and waited for the "perfect wave."

After several smaller waves washed over us, Jack looked over his shoulder and yelled: "Here comes a big one! Start paddling! Hard!"

In spite of my best efforts, the huge wave washed over me, knocking me off my board. As I reclaimed my perch, I saw Jack about 50 yards in front of me, riding the crest of that giant wave. He was standing on his board like a native as the wave pushed him toward the beach.

In spite of Jack's patient instructions, I didn't have the upper-body strength to get up enough speed to equal the wave's momentum. So, I never caught a wave, perfect or otherwise. I could now partially understand why Jack's chest and back muscles were so well-developed.

For the rest of the afternoon, no matter how hard I paddled, the results were always the same: Jack caught the wave that washed me off my board.

A couple of days later, Jack asked me to go with him to see the movie, "For Whom the Bell Tolls." Of course, I was delighted not only to be with Jack, but I was relieved that I wouldn't be competing with the Pacific Ocean again. Also, I had recently read Hemingway's novel in my English literature class. During one of the hospital scenes, Jack reached over and took my hand. After holding it gently for several minutes, he released it discreetly. I had forgotten to tell him that I suffered from sweaty palms.

On the way home, his car radio played softly as we rehashed the Spanish Civil war. He turned up the volume when a female voice began singing. We listened quietly until she had finished. I broke the silence: "I think I've heard that before. Do you know what it is?"

"Yes, I do. I made my operatic debut when I was thirteen singing with the lady we just heard in that same opera."

"Oh, you're kidding!"

"I'm serious. That was Risë Stevens singing the 'Habañera' from *Carmen*."

"Well, I've heard of her."

"My music teacher sang in the chorus of the San Antonio

Grand Opera Festival. She volunteered our music class to be the children's chorus in the opera."

"But that's in a foreign language, isn't it?"

"Yeah, French."

"Do you still remember any of it?"

"Let's see," Jack began, wrinkling his brow in thought. "We were playing a group of street urchins. We marched on stage in the first act mimicking the changing of the guard. It went like this:

Avec la garde montante.
Nous arrivons, nous voilà . . .
Sonne, trompette éclatante,
Ta-ra ta ta, ta-ra ta ta;
[We've come with the new guard,
We're arrived, we're here!
Blow, loud trumpets:
Ta-ra ta ta ta-ra ta ta.]"

"You seem to know a lot about opera," I volunteered, trying to continue the conversation.

"I fell in love with opera and Risë Stevens at the same time in 1946. Opera has sort of been my hobby ever since."

Jack and I saw each other several more times before my six weeks in paradise ended. At the airport, he gave me the traditional aloha kiss as he slipped the flower lei over my head. "Here's my address. Drop me a note when you have time," Jack said as Mother and I boarded the plane.

After takeoff, I heard Mother weeping softly. "Why are you crying, Mother?"

"I just hate to leave them, especially that baby," she sobbed.

"I don't know what you're crying about. You'll see them in a year. But I'll probably never see Jack Walker again," I remarked unsympathetically.

"Well, if you're interested, why don't you write him," she advised. "You never know what might happen."

Chapter Nine

Soothing relief spread over my body instantaneously, even before Mrs. Collins pulled out her morphine syringe.

It had been a long night for me. That all-too-familiar pain I had felt for the past several months hit me with a vengeance again during the early morning hours. It felt like the cancer was gnawing away at my bone.

With my pain eased, I drifted off to sleep immediately. Several hours later, I was awakened by Jack's kiss and greeting.

"Well, Sleeping Beauty, you're really sawing logs."

I looked at him blurredly with one eye. When I told him about my pain attack, he said he would continue to talk until I could clear my head from the deep sleep induced by the morphine. As he talked about home and the children, I noticed that in spite of his smiling face, his eyes looked tired. His face also looked thinner than I had remembered.

"How've you been feeling?" I began, by now awake enough to talk.

"Oh, fine," Jack responded characteristically. "But, your mother and sister have been begging to come to Maryland to see you."

"I wanted them to wait until I got home from the hospital so I could spend more time with them. What do you think?"

"Well, it will soon be six weeks that you've been in the hospital," Jack added. "I've been able to handle the kids, the house, and my job pretty well so far. The physical part just takes time. But it's the psychological part that's so difficult."

"I guess we really don't know how much longer I'll be in the hospital. So I think we should go ahead and tell them to make plans to come," I concluded as I looked at Jack's weary face.

"It'll be good to have some adult conversation at home for a change. And I could use some moral support about now, too."

"Don't worry, Mother and Jean will provide you with plenty of conversation," I laughed. "When do you suppose I'll get to see the kids? It's been such a long time."

"Just as soon as they'll let you. Why don't you try to arrange something with the doctor, and then I'll bring them up as soon as you get the green light."

In 1974 military hospitals did not allow children under twelve to visit wards. And I had not been allowed to get into a wheelchair to leave the ward since my admission.

As Jack ended his visit and left to go home to pick up the kids, I suddenly realized how selfish and inconsiderate I'd been. It was obvious that Jack needed family support. The poor guy had been on a treadmill for six weeks. I was only thinking of myself and what I wanted concerning my mother and sister.

I am truly convinced of the veracity of the old adage that it is often harder for those who stand and wait. Of one thing I am absolutely certain: I am the luckiest person in the world to have found and married Jack, whom I adore and who has stuck with me unstintingly through every adversity.

The Sunday before Valentine's Day turned out to be one of the most memorable of my hospital stay. Even though I still could not sit up in a wheelchair, I obtained permission from Dr. Slimmons to leave the ward on a gurney to visit Jack and the children in the patients' lounge. When I made my grand entrance, David and Amy ran to greet me with hugs and kisses. Jack had dressed them in their Sunday best, and they looked great. I spent the next couple of hours catching up on school activities and helping the children address valentines to all of their classmates. That Sunday really turned out to be a sweetheart of a day.

My long-awaited rendezvous with radiation therapy was scheduled for the next day. By the time Jack arrived, I had already transferred to a gurney. As he pushed me through the corridors en route to the radiation clinic, we chatted apprehensively about the upcoming treatments, which could mean the difference between life and death. After a short wait, I was summoned by a voice coming from a huge frame which seemed to fill the doorway. The source of that voice was Dr. Beatty, a Paul Bunyan lookalike with a full, reddish beard. All he lacked to make the comparison complete was an ax and "Babe."

Dr. Beatty bubbled with self-confidence and enthusiasm as he briefed us on the physical principles and marvels of radiation therapy. The only thing I comprehended was the part about radiation destroying malignant cells at a rate far greater than healthy cells.

This stimulated Jack's curiosity. "What about her porous bone?"

"Once the malignant cells are killed off, the bone should regenerate and fill in," Dr. Beatty continued his praise of his chosen specialty.

Jack was still curious. "Does radiation therapy have a pretty good success rate?"

"Yes, indeed," Dr. Beatty nodded as he began measuring the length of my thigh bone. "We've had good success against Hodgkin's disease. And that's a kissing cousin to your type of cancer."

After considerable further explanations, Dr. Beatty exuberantly asked, "How about having the first treatment today?"

I looked at Jack as he turned to look at me. I summed up both our feelings: "Why not?"

Dr. Beatty rushed about taking more measurements and making calculations. He explained that they planned to radiate both of my femur bones completely, from the knee to the pelvis, front and back. He also figured the number of units of absorbed radiation dose, or "rads," my body could take. By his calculations, I needed daily treatments for six weeks.

Pulling my hospital gown aside, Dr. Beatty tediously began drawing lines with a red indelible marker on the top part of my thigh, outlining the femur bone. He did this on both legs. He explained how they would use these lines to arrange lead shields in the machine to protect surrounding tissue from the devastation of the radiation beam. Then, with Jack's help, he turned me over to complete the therapeutic road map on the reverse side. What a strange sensation to lie on my stomach again after lying flat on my back for six weeks!

When he had completed his artistic handiwork, I commented facetiously: "If you ever get tired of this work, I'll bet you could get a job with Rand McNally."

After almost two hours of preparation and briefing, I was now ready for my first treatment. We descended by elevator to the lower level of a large room and entered a smaller room which resembled a bank vault, complete with a heavy lead-lined door. Dr. Beatty and Jack transferred me to a table in the middle of the room. I was lying directly beneath a huge device which was quite reminiscent of the grain silos back in Iowa. Dr. Beatty explained that his machine was one of the original radiation equipments installed in the United States. And although it may look antiquated, it was still quite efficient in doing what it was supposed to do.

When he had completed arranging the light beam on the red marks on my legs, Dr. Beatty and Jack left the room. As the huge door swung shut behind them, I was overwhelmed by the complete silence surrounding me. No Egyptian tomb was ever more silent or engulfing. I felt a little bit like the title character in Aïda where, in the final scene, she chooses to be entombed alive with her lover, Rhadames. On second thought, I reasoned, Aïda had her lover with her, but my lover was outside my "tomb" with Dr. Beatty. My plight was more like the heroine in *Manon Lescaut*. Like Manon, I was "*sola, perduta, abbandonata. . .* [alone, lost, and abandoned.]"

"Hold still, Mary! Don't move!" Dr. Beatty's voice bellowed from a speaker in the corner of the room, ending my operatic musing. "We're watching you on closed circuit television to make sure you're okay."

"Do I have to hold my breath like in other X-rays?"

"No. You'd be hard pressed to do that for twenty minutes. Just don't move."

The actual radiation treatments, which became my daily routine for the next six weeks, turned out to be painless. However, after about the first ten days, the center of my legs turned a brilliant red. It was like the worst case of sunburn I ever had. The burn was especially bad on the back of my legs extending up to the buttocks, an area not normally exposed to the sun. My skin ultimately burned and peeled several times during the treatment period. Since I was not allowed to use any lotions or oils on the treatment days, the only relief I had was on weekends when I could treat the burns with lotion. Even though my legs looked the color of a boiled lobster, Dr. Beatty was right. The radiation *was* killing the cancer cells because I never had a recurrence of the excruciating bone pain after my first treatment.

Jean and Mother arrived within days of each other. Coming from Minneapolis, Mother was well prepared for winter weather. But Jean's Arizona wardrobe was a bit scanty for a Washington February.

Jean, my only sibling, is a full-of-life, fun-loving person. Although as children we had our differences because of her four-year age advantage, as adults I consider her one of my best friends. Almost everyone agrees that we share certain family physical characteristics such as hair texture, voice quality, and complexion. These traits were poignantly brought home to Jean one night shortly after she arrived while she was bathing the children. They told her that she sounded just like their Mom.

My mother's and sister's visit was a godsend for Jack. He could now devote more time to his job and not have to worry about who would meet the kids after school. But more importantly to him, after weeks of bearing the mental anguish of my illness alone, he now had, at least temporarily, loving family members to help share his burdens.

CHAPTER TEN

My sister's two-week stay passed quickly. My mother and Jean arrived at my hospital room each day just before lunch carrying their meal so we could all eat together. We shared lots of conversation, some humorous and some very touching.

All of us were in tears when Jean told us about helping Jack the previous day with some house cleaning. This had been her first visit to our house, and naturally she was admiring some of the art objects we had collected from different parts of the world. She was particularly impressed with a blue, antique German beer stein with the date "1720" engraved on the pewter top. When she was speculating about the monetary value of such a rare piece, Jack told her that all his material possessions meant nothing to him without Mary to share them. She also asked Jack why the door to the family room had been closed ever since her arrival. He replied that that was the room in which he and Mary had shared so much happiness together in the past, and that he had closed the door New Year's night because he couldn't bear being in there alone.

In a lighter vein, I was in stitches (in more ways than one) when Mother and Jean recounted their toboggan run down interstate highway 70S (now I.H. 270) from Rockville to Bethesda with Lou Ponder driving his new, front-wheel-drive Cadillac. It had snowed about eight inches, which, for the Washington, D.C. area, was tantamount to a blizzard. But Lou was not one to be intimidated by the weather or anything else, and he insisted that Mother, Jean, Jack, and the children join him and Hilda for dinner at his favorite Chinese restaurant. Most of the government workers had been released early that day, and a snow emergency was in effect. That meant snow tires or chains were mandatory for all vehicles on public roads. Like most "southern" cities, Washington and its suburbs are never prepared for snow, and no snowplow had yet ventured into our part of the metropolitan area. Everyone piled into Lou's car, and off they mushed. When they got on the interstate highway, it was obvious that even that main artery had not been plowed. Dozens of cars dotted the roadside, stuck in snow drifts and abandoned or stalled from mechanical problems. One lane in each direction of the four-lane divided highway had been packed down from a continuous line of slow-moving traffic throughout the afternoon. Lou was not having any of that. He abruptly turned over into the snow-filled lane, passing the slower-moving traffic as though it was standing still. At times, he accelerated up to 70 miles per hour, hurling the snow to the left and right like a supersonic snow blower. Jean said David relished every moment of this snowy odyssey, but Jack sat as transfixed as an ice sculpture.

I was still receiving my daily radiation treatments, and each afternoon my mother and sister eagerly volunteered to chauffeur me to and from my lead-lined sanctuary. Hospital gurneys maneuver about like a Mack truck, and with the distaff members of the Crawford family at the controls, it was a thrill a minute.

By the time my treatment was over and Mother and Jean had wheeled me back to my room, Jack was either waiting or had arrived simultaneously to begin his daily visit. Mother and Jean usually left for home about that time to be with David and Amy and to start dinner.

Needless to say, these three visitors, plus David and Amy on Sundays, were the highlight of my day during those weeks. Throughout my initial couple of weeks in the hospital, I was practically inundated with visitors. Friends, acquaintances, and consulting physicians visited in such profusion that I practically had to have a reservation to use the bedpan. But when the diagnosis of cancer became known, the visitors began to dwindle over time. By the sixth or seventh week it became obvious who our "real" friends were. Jack and I discussed this phenomenon several times, and we attributed it to a combination of reasons. I had become a "new leper" in the minds of certain individuals. For some, it may have been because they felt uncomfortable around me and didn't quite know what to say. For others, we got the distinct impression that they were fearful of "catching" my dreaded disease. But our true friends remained undaunted by the fear, ignorance, or prejudice shown by a few, and we treasure those friendships to this day.

I had been pestering Dr. Slimmons for the past week to allow me to go home for a trial weekend. Although I still couldn't stand, I was now able to transfer to a wheelchair. His first reaction was skepticism about my ability to function away from the hospital this soon, even with help from Jack, Mother, and Jean. I guess I finally wore him down, because during his evening rounds on the Thursday before the weekend, he finally acquiesced. I was so ecstatic that I called Jack at his office to share the good news. About an hour later, Jack showed up grinning from ear to ear. He was carrying a quart of ice cream.

"This is in celebration of your homecoming." He gave a mischievous laugh as he began opening the package.

"What flavor is it?" I asked cautiously.

"Your favorite! Licorice!"

Jack knew that licorice ice cream would remind me of the rather bizarre encounter we had with this flavor during a snowy Christmas holiday in Minnesota in the winter of 1958.

I had accepted the advice Mother offered me as we were leaving Hawaii, and I wrote a brief, newsy note to Jack shortly after we arrived back on the mainland.

Within a few days, I received a long, thoughtfully written letter from Jack. I knew he had graduated with honors in journalism from The University of Texas, but I had never known anyone before who wrote philosophical letters. I answered his letter with some trepidation, fearing my folksy prose would brand me as a hick from Minnesota. But apparently Jack looked beyond my sentence structure to something more elusive because his next letter arrived even more promptly than his first. Thus began what was to become a romance by mail.

It was amazing to me how much better we got to know each other over the next three months based solely on our letters. Since I was still in college, Jack had more time for writing than I had.

By the time November arrived, Jack was averaging three letters a week, while I was lucky to find time to send one or two.

At Thanksgiving Jack wrote to let me know he was planning a trip home at Christmas to visit his parents. He asked if he could come via Minneapolis to visit me and to meet my Dad. After getting the green light from my folks, it didn't take long for me to decide to invite him to spend Christmas with us.

Jack's plane was delayed in Seattle due to heavy fog, and he arrived in Minneapolis about 8 p.m. on the Sunday before Christmas, about three hours late.

As Jack deplaned, my parents and I noticed that he was wearing his Navy raincoat, without the insignia, and was bare-headed. His bronzed skin stood out in contrast to the pale, sun-deprived Minnesotans around us. Jack greeted Mom and me with a Hawaiian flower lei and a kiss. Then I introduced him to Dad. There seemed to be an instant rapport between the two men. Whatever apprehensions Jack may have felt about meeting Dad under these circumstances seemed to disappear as soon as Dad welcomed him.

My Dad, Dave Crawford, was a gentle, outgoing person who never met a stranger. His affection for his family knew no bounds. There was absolutely nothing he wouldn't do for us. Although not much taller than Jack, he seemed to me to be a giant of a man. Always a tease, he was a witty individual whom my sister and I affectionately called "Scrooge" in the Gilbertian sense, which was the exact opposite of his generous nature.

As we walked toward our car in the brisk, night air, I noticed Jack was shivering.

"I guess this weather is a little different from what you left in Hawaii," I laughed.

"I'll say it is," Jack muttered through chattering teeth. "When I left Honolulu it was 80 degrees. How cold is it here?"

"It's not too bad," Dad interjected. "It's only about ten below zero."

"I've never been in below zero weather before," Jack shuddered. "I feel like someone has put a clamp on my nose!"

As we made our way out of the airport parking lot past the dirty piles of snow steeped up head high along the roadway, Dad suggested that we go home via downtown Minneapolis to see the animated department store windows.

Dad parked the car near Dayton's Department Store, and the four of us began walking like excited school kids along Hennepen Avenue, "oohing" and "aahing" at the Christmas fantasies behind the glass.

After strolling for about 30 minutes on the frozen pavement, I noticed Jack's lips were almost purple. Dad took his cue from me and suggested that we go to Bridgeman's for a snack.

Jack happily agreed to go anywhere to get out of the piercing cold. As we walked into Bridgeman's, his expression turned to disbelief as he discovered Bridgeman's was an ice-cream parlor.

Mom and Dad ordered their usual flavors. I ordered my all-time favorite ice-cream flavor—licorice.

"Licorice?" Jack asked incredulously.

"Oh, it's great! You've got to try it!" I suggested.

"I think I'll just have plain vanilla," Jack muttered, his lips still numbed by the cold.

In retrospect, Jack must have thought that the harsh Minnesota winter had frozen our brains to top off a stroll down the avenue in ten-below-zero weather with a trip to an ice-cream parlor.

The remaining few days before Christmas, my favorite holiday of the year, flew by quickly with last-minute shopping, sightseeing, and introducing Jack to my friends. More importantly, Jack and I were getting to know each other better.

On Christmas Eve, Jack asked if it would be possible to watch Menotti's opera, *Amahl and the Night Visitors*, on television. It was then that I learned the true extent of Jack's interest in opera.

"You really do like opera, don't you Jack?" I observed, trying to show interest in an area with which I was only vaguely familiar.

"I don't just *like* opera, Mary. I *love* it! To me opera is almost like a religious experience."

"That sounds sacrilegious," I noted.

"I know," he continued, "and I didn't intend it to be. What I'm trying to say—and this isn't easy to articulate—is that opera occupies a special pinnacle in the artistic world. Great paintings give the viewer an aesthetic thrill, stirring symphonies move our emotions, and noble poetry goes straight to the heart. But opera does all of those things and much more. It can be spine-tingling in its beauty and hair-raising in its dramatic impact. When an art form does that, it stops being a means of entertainment and becomes an uplifting, almost sublime, experience."

"Wow! You really are serious about opera," I said, in obvious understatement. "I like some classical music and Broadway musicals. But, to me, they are just entertainment."

"I know. I like Broadway too. But I'm talking about an intensified world which blends music, words, vocal sound, visual art, drama, spectacle, and, at times, dance to produce an experience without equal. Great opera can awaken the soul, ennoble it, and move it to the highest levels of human experience."

After several seconds of thoughtful reflection, I finally broke the silence: "I'm not sure I'm capable of ever loving opera that much."

"You may not be. But I bet you are," he replied. "I didn't just start out with the same level of understanding and appreciation that I have today. It's taken years of work and study. But you have to make an investment in time and effort. All I can say is that it's the best investment I've ever made."

Shortly after the music began, Dad promptly fell asleep and began snoring. This was my first exposure to a complete opera, and I was surprised that I enjoyed it.

"Wake up, Dad, it's almost time to go to church services," I called as I turned off the television. Dad slowly opened his eyes.

"How did you like the opera, Honey?" Mom laughed.

"That 'A-mule' was really something," Dad replied knowingly.

We never let Dad know that we knew he hadn't heard any of it.

Christmas Day 1958 turned out to be a banner day. Jack gave me a beautiful solitaire pearl ring, mounted in brilliant gold, that he had purchased in Japan. After a busy day, Mom and Dad went to bed early. Jack and I sat around the Christmas tree, basking in the warmth and radiance of the day. The attraction that I had felt toward Jack since our first meeting in Hawaii had grown steadily since July. His presence around me during this Christmas season seemed almost magical. Could he be the man of my destiny who I had dreamed of and yearned for all my life? I had never known true love before, so I wasn't sure if that dull glow in my heart meant this was the "real thing" or not. Jack's sentiments apparently mirrored mine as he began to declare his feelings toward me. A lot of tender moments were expressed and felt, so I wasn't surprised when he declared his love and asked me to marry him. As much as I loved Jack, I didn't give him a positive response until the next morning after I had discussed his proposal with my parents. I didn't think they would object, but I wanted to give them the courtesy of discussing his proposal with them before I said yes. That seems pretty old-fashioned today, but I loved and respected my parents so much that I wouldn't have done anything to hurt them.

Jack probably didn't sleep much that night after getting up

The Fat Lady Hasn't Sung

enough courage to pop the question only to have me put the answer on hold for the next eight hours. But we were both ecstatic the next morning when I gave him my answer. I suggested that we use the pearl ring he had given me for Christmas as an engagement ring. But Jack was too much of a traditionalist for that. So the next day we went shopping for a diamond ring to signify our love and betrothal. We picked out a beautiful half carat, solitaire-mounted diamond ring. To this day, it is the most gorgeous ring I've ever seen.

The rest of Jack's visit seemed even more magical than the first part. We planned a June wedding to be held after my graduation and, hopefully, coincidental with Jack's permanent change of station orders from the Navy.

Jack boarded a plane for Texas the day after New Year's. He spent about a week with his parents before returning to Hawaii. The day after his departure, he wrote what was to be the first in a series of love letters. He composed a letter each day, seven days a week, right up until he returned for the wedding in June. What letters! He expressed his love so poetically in so many different ways! I believe he must have been inspired by Elizabeth Barrett Browning's immortal words: "How do I love thee? Let me count the ways."

The Navy cooperated nicely with our plans, and we were able to set the twentieth of June, 1959, as our wedding date, during Jack's transfer from Hawaii to Washington, D.C.

We were married in a twilight ceremony in the Edina, Minnesota Colonial Church. It was a lovely double-ring ceremony in a chapel with nosegays decorating each pew. Inscribed inside both wedding rings were the Hawaiian words *Manawa Pau Kau*. Translated roughly, that means "always yours." I thought how appropriate that phrase was as I took the vows which made me the wife of Lieutenant Jack O. Walker, U.S. Navy.

Chapter Eleven

Trial week-end or not, coming home after eight weeks in the hospital was even better than I imagined. As I wheeled out into the sparkling sunlight, it seemed as though I was experiencing the world for the first time. Everything appeared to me magnified and brighter than I remembered it. Even though the trees were still bare, there was a slight hint of spring in the air.

Because I was still unable to bear any weight on my legs, it was necessary to use a transfer board to form a bridge to move from wheelchair, to car, to bed, or another chair. My transfer board was about three feet long, eight inches wide, and made of hardwood. Multiple coats of varnish gave it a mirror-like sheen. When I moved along the board, I felt like a kid again on a slide.

As we pulled into the driveway, Mom, Jean, and the kids came out to greet me. It seemed like it had been such a long time since I left the house on that cold, damp, New Year's day. But to me, like Rhadames, this was a triumphal return. It was obvious upon entering the house that everyone had been busy preparing for my homecoming. The family room downstairs had been converted into a bedroom and outfitted with all my medical necessities, including a commode chair which Jack had rented.

Even though the weekend went too fast, I convinced everyone that I could function at home. I knew then that my remaining days at Bethesda were numbered. As I headed back to the hospital Sunday night, Jean was winging her way home to Arizona.

My last two weeks in the hospital continued the routine which had been established earlier. However, in addition to my daily radiation treatments, light physical therapy was added. I looked forward to these trips to the PT clinic, not only for the change in routine, but because of the professional staff and the upbeat patients.

At that time wounded veterans of the Vietnam War were still being treated at Bethesda. Two of those veterans were Steve and Larry. We ended up sharing a common mat for our daily workouts.

Steve had an athletic body with a head of close-cropped blonde hair which topped his thick, muscular neck. The pant legs of his pajama bottoms were knotted just below his pelvis to accommodate the void where his legs had once been.

Larry, by contrast, was tall and thin, with dark curly hair. He was missing the bottom half of his left leg. Both of these young men had encountered land mines in separate incidents. In spite of their devastating loss, I was constantly amazed at their lack of bitterness and at their positive attitude.

"Hey, Mary, we've got a spot for you over here," Steve yelled.

"We've got some hot coffee for you to get your engine started," Larry grinned.

I wheeled over to my "reserved" spot and transferred on to the mat.

"I've heard of 'going to the mat' with someone, but this is ridiculous," I laughed as I picked up my barbell.

After several minutes of exercising, Larry suggested a coffee break. He told us this was the day he was going to have his final fitting for his prosthesis.

"Now you'll be able to tap dance through life," Steve joked.

"Knock it off, Steve, or I'll beat you with my stump."

"Are they going to be able to fit you for a prosthesis, Steve," I inquired.

"No, I won't be able to walk again. But I just thank God that the mine wasn't any closer or I'd be singing soprano today," Steve added without any touch of rancor.

The physical therapist interrupted our break with her pat phrase. "Back to work you three! No pain, no gain!"

To this day I still remember how Steve and Larry taught me to "pop wheelies" in my wheelchair, much to Jack's chagrin.

During my time in the hospital, I had been checking periodically on Barbara Brown's condition. She had remained in a vegetative state for the three months since her stroke. As I wheeled myself back to the orthopedic ward, I was surprised to see Barbara's husband, Ben, waiting outside my door.

"Hi, Ben! How's Barbara doing?"

Ben looked up sadly. The strain of the last several months was etched in his face. "Barbara passed away this morning, Mary. I knew you would want to know."

As I tried to console Ben, it was difficult for me to believe that Barbara, that vibrant, self-assured woman, was gone.

A couple of days before my discharge from the hospital, Jack and I met with Dr. Perlin to discuss his plans for my upcoming chemotherapy treatments. Jack maneuvered my wheelchair carefully into his cluttered office, piled high with medical books and files.

"You'll be finishing your radiation treatments in a couple of weeks. Our plan is to start your chemotherapy treatments immediately thereafter," Dr. Perlin spoke softly, peering over the top of his glasses. "Since this is your first experience with chemotherapy, I thought you'd like to know a little about how it works."

"I'm anxious to know what to expect," I replied.

Dr. Perlin explained how chemotherapy is one of the three major tools in fighting cancer. The other two are surgery and radiation. Chemotherapy not only kills malignant cells, but it also destroys normal cells. There are numerous "recipes" combining various drugs that are used to fight different types of cancer.

"We have decided to use Cytoxin, Oncovin, and Prednisone for your type of cancer."

"Will there be any side effects?" I inquired.

"All chemotherapy drugs have potential side effects. With these particular drugs, you may experience nausea, body aches, and loss of hair among others."

"Will I get this by injection or what?"

"This particular protocol will be taken orally for three days. Then you'll have a three-week rest before you have the next dose."

"When do you plan to start?" Jack interjected.

"The Monday following Mary's last radiation treatment."

Happily, Dr. Slimmons didn't change his mind about discharging me, and I was released the next day with many admonitions to be careful.

It was wonderful knowing that this trip home was for real and not on a trial basis.

My first morning home I was awakened by a loud hammering noise.

"What on earth is going on, Honey?" I yelled to Jack as he bounded down the stairs.

"I don't know, but I'm sure as hell going to find out," he said as he hurriedly unlocked the front door.

Much to Jack's relief, the source of the noise wasn't hostile.

Lou Ponder was standing next to a pile of lumber, and his carpenter friend, Richard, was building a frame on our front porch.

"Come on in, Lou. We're just getting up. How about some coffee?" I heard Jack say.

"We'll have some coffee later," Lou replied, puffing on his ever-present cigarette. "In case you're wondering what's going on, we're building a ramp for Mary's wheelchair."

Even though Jack tried several times to pay for Richard's time and materials, Lou always refused, saying it was a welcome home gift.

The last two weeks of radiation treatments flew by. The skin on my legs was now lobster red. I had received the maximum dose of radiation for my body weight, and it felt like it.

With Easter nearing, we were all anxiously awaiting a week's visit from Dad. It had been the previous Easter since we had seen him. Jack and I had driven to Minneapolis with the kids over the Easter holidays the year before and had a great time. Mom and Dad had rented a room for us at a nearby hotel which boasted an indoor swimming pool. David obviously had been exposed to chicken pox earlier, because two days before we had planned to come home, he broke out with the first visible skin eruptions. By the time we started our return drive, he had a full-blown case of the disease. Although his face and body were covered by the blemishes, his appetite was unaffected. Meal times on the trip home were always a challenge because Jack and I would have to think of ingenious ways to sneak David into restaurants without drawing attention to his pox. We probably spread the chicken pox virus from Minneapolis to Rockville during those two days of travel.

Our next weekend was a tale of two emotions. On the one hand, I was jubilant about Dad's arrival for a week's visit. Conversely, I approached my upcoming chemotherapy sessions with great trepidation.

Dad arrived as scheduled on Saturday, and Jack began a week's leave so he could be with us during my first chemotherapy.

Early Monday morning Jack and I reported to Dr. Perlin's office. My initial chemotherapy dosage already had been counted out and was waiting for me. There were 27 pills each of Cytoxin, Oncovin, and Prednisone in very large milligram tablets. Dr. Perlin methodically explained that I should take three pills of each type, three times a day for three days. He suggested taking them immediately after eating in order to minimize nausea.

We made a point of staying pretty close to home those first few days, not because I was sick, but because we were unsure of my possible reaction to the drugs.

Based on my initial tolerance for the chemicals, Jack suggested that as a celebration for completing my first regimen that we all go to the Ringling Bros. & Barnum and Bailey Circus on Saturday in Washington.

By the time I swallowed the last of my pills on Wednesday night, I was still feeling pretty well. I felt a bit queasy by then, and my appetite, never large, had just about vanished.

But things started changing on Thursday. By noon, my entire body ached as if I had been squeezed by a huge vise. It was like the ache of having the flu, magnified a thousand times. The skin on every part of my body was hypersensitive to the touch. My mouth had the taste of mildew even after brushing my teeth.

As nightfall descended, it was obvious that I wasn't getting any better. The aching racked my entire body.

Watching my distress, Jack decided to do something to help me. He pulled a telephone book out of a drawer and began looking for a number. He quickly found what he was looking for and began dialing.

I could hear his conversation with Dr. Perlin. Jack told him about my reaction to the chemotherapy and asked if I could take aspirin to help relieve my aches. Dr. Perlin readily agreed, and within a few seconds Jack brought me some relief.

Most of my body aches had subsided by Saturday, and our trip to the circus, somewhat in question earlier, was all set again.

The arena in Washington, like many older buildings, was too old to have wheelchair access. Therefore, we persuaded the circus management to let us sit right up front on the main floor in front of the first row of permanent seats. We were, of course, treated to one of the most lavishly beautiful spectacles imaginable. David and Amy were enthralled by the entire performance. The highlight of the show for Amy came when Gunther Gebel-Williams, the famous animal trainer, picked up Amy and gave her a ride around the arena on his white horse. It was love at first ride. This experience probably marked the beginning of Amy's life-long interest in horses.

Although I felt reasonably well under the circumstances, Jack repeatedly asked me how I was feeling. He commented each time how pale I looked.

Late the next day Dad caught his return flight to Minneapolis. I felt a little guilty about him using a week of his vacation time to sit around and watch me ache.

Jack's leave also had expired, and he returned to work on Monday morning. When he came home that evening, he commented again on my ashen countenance. I assured him I was feeling fine.

But I was still tired from my first week of chemotherapy, and I was more than ready to go to bed after watching the news.

Early Tuesday morning, about sunrise, I awoke feeling terribly light-headed. I struggled to move my body across the sheets to the commode chair parked and locked in place next to my bed. The room seemed to be spinning, and I thought that, with such dizziness and diarrhea, I must have picked up a virus at the circus.

As the dizziness intensified, I figured I'd better get some help since I wasn't sure I could make it back onto the bed without assistance. Since Jack and Mom were sleeping in the upstairs bedrooms, I didn't think my cries for help could be heard in my weakened condition. So, I summoned forth my most reliable noisemaker—my famous whistle. I whistled through my teeth and called Jack's name as loudly as I could. Immediately after uttering his name, I passed out.

Jack isn't sure what woke him, my whistle and shouts or his alarm, but, true to his usual practice, he immediately headed down the stairs to check on me.

After I fainted, I apparently slumped forward and onto the bed. Jack's frantic shouts of my name apparently awakened my mother, and she also was downstairs within seconds.

Dark brown-colored blood covered my commode chair and bed since I had lost control during my unconscious state.

I regained consciousness from time to time and heard Jack calling EMS. Mother was applying wet towels to my head and trying to clean me up before the ambulance arrived.

In less than 20 minutes from the time Jack found me, I was loaded aboard the vehicle.

The siren wailed and the lights flashed as we headed south on

The Fat Lady Hasn't Sung

Interstate 70S toward Bethesda Naval Hospital. The ambulance bypassed most of the bumper-to-bumper rush-hour traffic by using the shoulder of the highway.

I drifted in and out of consciousness during the journey. But each time I came to, I saw Jack's face near me and felt his hand holding mine.

Chapter Twelve

"My God, where is all her blood? She has no count!"

"That's what we're trying to find out, Dr. Perlin," the emergency room doctor answered curtly as he and several other medical people frantically hovered over me trying to start an i.v.

Those were the first words I recall hearing after my arrival at the emergency room.

As soon as the EMS ambulance reached Bethesda, Dr. Perlin, as my oncologist of record, was summoned. He had ordered a CBC (complete blood count) and had requested an emergency typing and cross-matching of my blood. His bewildering question was in response to the reports he had just received from the laboratory.

Dr. Perlin ordered the emergency room staff to begin a blood transfusion immediately. It seemed that within minutes after the new blood began coursing through my veins, my weakness and light-headedness began to subside. At least now I was able to maintain consciousness and realize Jack and Mother were waiting nearby. Mother had followed the ambulance in our car so she and Jack would have a way to get home later.

Since the blood had been refrigerated until just before my transfusion, it was still quite cold. It wasn't long before my whole body felt thoroughly chilled, and I remember shivering even with a blanket covering me.

After receiving another batch of reports from the lab, Dr. Perlin approached me.

"Mary, it's obvious to us that you're bleeding internally. They can't do anything else here in the emergency room. So, I've made arrangements to admit you to the internal medicine ward."

"Do you have any idea what the source of the bleeding is?" I asked.

"Not at this time. But I'm going to order a series of tests to try and find out."

When I arrived on the ward, accompanied by Jack and Mom, I was met by two young, white-coated staff members.

"Mrs. Walker, I'm Dr. Volpe, and this is my associate, Dr. Weaver," the smaller of the two men began. "Dr. Perlin has assigned us to be your personal physicians during your tests."

I couldn't believe that those two baby-faced guys were doctors. However, I felt reassured that they had to know something since they had probably just finished reading their medical books last week.

As we struggled to transfer me to the bed, I noticed something was missing.

"This sure would be a lot easier with a 'monkey-bar,'" I sighed as I wrestled to protect my i.v. lines.

"What are 'monkey-bars?'" the interns asked in unison.

"You know, that's what all the orthopedic patients swing on." I then described the trapeze-like bar that is suspended over the top of a bed and is used to help immobile patients transfer.

"Before you leave, would you please send someone in with a bed pan?" I asked.

After the doctors left, I noticed Jack and Mom looked terribly concerned.

"Don't be worried, you two. I know they'll get to the bottom of this."

"I think I'd better call Dad," Mom said in a trembling voice.

"No, let's wait and see what we find out. He just got home," I replied confidently.

Dr. Volpe reappeared with a fresh unit of blood.

"You're still bleeding heavily, Mrs. Walker. We're going to continue with the transfusions until we solve the problem. You have your first test right after lunch."

The two doctors arrived about 12:30 pulling a gurney.

"Okay, Mrs. Walker. We're going to be your pilot and co-pilot through these tests," Dr. Weaver smiled.

"*You* are going to be push-me, pull-me?" I asked, looking surprised. "Gee, I didn't know you were Dr. Doolittle. Can you explain why I'm getting such high-priced gurney pushers?"

"Yes, because we need to monitor your i.v. fluids and blood," Dr. Volpe replied.

"Where are we going first?" I questioned.

"To the scope room," Dr. Weaver responded.

"Oh, boy! Another appearance with the scope brothers— endo and procto," I said unenthusiastically.

The two doctors loaded me back on the gurney, and the three of us began our strange trek, rushing through the corridors of Bethesda.

The scope examinations hadn't gotten any better since my first exposure to those instruments of torture a few weeks earlier.

Just as we finished the last scope exam, a breathless corpsman carrying two blood-filled bags caught up with us.

"Thank goodness you made it on time," Dr. Volpe began. "We were about to run on fumes."

"I know," the flush-faced corpsman responded. "But I had to wait for the platelets to arrive."

"What in the world are platelets?" I interjected.

"They're elements of the blood which help start clotting," Dr. Weaver replied.

"So now you will be getting four different fluids—blood plasma, platelets, glucose solution, and antibiotics," Dr. Volpe said as he added the latest bags to my growing collection on the i.v. pole.

With bags flying, the two doctors rushed me off in the direction of the X-ray department. Upon our arrival, I wasn't surprised to find out I was scheduled for an upper and lower gastrointestinal (G.I.) series—a barium swallow and enema.

The first test was the upper G.I. The X-ray nurse offered me a choice of barium flavors—chocolate, vanilla, or strawberry. I chose strawberry, but it didn't do much for the chalky taste.

Needless to say, they didn't give me a choice of flavors for the enema.

After what seemed like an interminable time having radiologists pushing barium around to every nook and cranny in my torso, we finally finished up in X-ray about 6 p.m.

"How're you feeling, Mrs. Walker?" Dr. Volpe asked as we began heading back to my room.

"Like I was rode hard and put up wet!"

The two doctors were still chuckling as they pushed me into my room. I was delighted to see the "monkey-bar" in place over my bed.

"Oh great! Now I'll be able to transfer to my bed so much easier. I became pretty good at this during the months I spent in orthopedics. I even thought about applying for a position with the Flying Wallendas."

Although somewhat encumbered by all my life-lines, I swung onto my bed as the two doctors rolled their eyes in disbelief.

After eating dinner and watching TV for a while, I presumed I wouldn't see any of my doctors until morning.

About 9 p.m., however, Dr. Volpe showed up. He had a serious look on his face.

"Dr. Volpe," I began, "what are you doing here so late?"

"Oh, I had some work to catch up on. And I also wanted to talk to you."

"Have you received any of the reports from the tests?"

"I've got them all now."

"Did they show the source of the bleeding?"

"Unfortunately, nothing showed up. They were all normal.

So we're back to square one."

"What's our next plan of attack?"

Dr. Volpe checked my blood bottles. After a short pause he replied. "We're going to continue giving you more platelets in the hope that they will slow or stop the bleeding."

Dr. Volpe checked the i.v. lines and the tissue around the receiving vein in my arm. After a few moments, he continued. "I want to let you know that as a matter of policy we are putting you on the critical list. I need to let your husband know."

"Why don't you use my phone," I suggested. "Then I can talk to him after you're finished."

Dr. Volpe dialed the number I gave him, and I heard him talking to Jack. He explained that in cases such as mine, involving uncontrolled bleeding, such action was required. Dr. Volpe gave me the phone and said goodnight.

Jack seemed remarkably calm as I brought him up to date on the test results. He said he and Mom would be at the hospital shortly after lunch tomorrow.

Throughout the night I kept the staff busy replenishing my blood supply and i.v. fluids and emptying bed pans.

Early the next morning, I was awakened by Doctors Perlin, Volpe, and Weaver. They informed me that if the bleeding didn't slow down by noon, they were going to call in the surgeons to discuss options with me.

The rest of the morning was spent playing the waiting game. It also provided an opportunity for the nursing staff to catch up on my medical history.

Shortly after lunch, a man and a woman wearing white coats appeared.

"Mrs. Walker? I'm Dr. Scott, head of the blue surgical team. And this is my associate, Dr. Bach," the male half of the pair began. "We're here to discuss your situation and to let you know our thoughts on the problem."

As he talked, I noticed he had a generally disheveled look about him.

Dr. Scott continued. "From a surgical point of view, you have two options—exploratory surgery or the status quo."

"What would exploratory surgery entail?" I asked.

"We would have to examine all 26 feet of your intestines in the hope of finding the bleeder," Dr. Scott said.

"And the odds of finding it are not very favorable," Dr. Bach added in a fatalistic voice.

"What happens if you don't find it?" I asked apprehensively.

"You would bleed to death."

As Dr. Scott uttered those last few words, I again had the sensation that his words were coming from a great distance, reminiscent of my original cancer diagnosis.

Although I knew internal bleeding was serious, death this way had not entered my mind until I heard Dr. Scott use the "D" word. I guess Jack is right when he sometimes calls me a Pollyanna.

"And if I opt for the status quo, that is certain death?"

Dr. Scott's eyes did not make contact with mine as he spoke softly. "Ultimately, we would have to stop the blood transfusions, and the result would be the same."

"So I really don't have any option but surgery if I want to live?" I questioned, still trying to find a slim reed of hope.

Neither of the two doctors responded.

After several seconds of silence, my decision was clear. "Let's go with the exploratory surgery! Will the two of you be performing the operation?"

"No, the operating room is completely booked for today," Dr. Scott answered. "Your procedure will have to be done after hours by the surgical on-call team on duty for tonight."

The two doctors hadn't been gone long when Jack looked around the corner of the door, smiled at me, and said, "I've got a surprise for you, Mary, darlin'!"

Before I could ask what it was, I saw Dad coming through the door with Mom in tow.

"What are you doing here, Dad? You didn't even have time to unpack."

"Oh, I thought I'd work on my frequent flyer points," Dad

laughed as he embraced me.

Even though I hated to have Dad return so quickly, it was great to have my three greatest boosters with me at this time.

With my i.v. bottles running on high, I spent the next couple of hours bringing Jack, Mom, and Dad up to date on all my test results. I told them about my upcoming exploratory surgery, but I was careful to omit the discussion with Dr. Scott on my survival chances. I felt there was no need to worry them needlessly.

Dr. Volpe returned with a fresh unit of blood and placed it piggy-back on the previous unit. He was closely followed by Doctors Scott and Bach who were escorting a familiar face—Dr. Gregory.

I was ecstatic to learn that this self-assured surgeon, who had so skillfully performed my thyroid surgery, would be heading the emergency team for my operation.

Dr. Gregory complimented Dr. Volpe for having prepared me so thoroughly for the surgery. He then gave the four of us a short briefing on some of the details of the upcoming procedure. As he departed to scrub and get his team ready, he said he would see me in about 30 minutes.

Jack followed the doctors into the hall. As I learned later, he privately asked Dr. Scott some of the same questions I had raised earlier. He got the same answers I did.

After I transferred to a gurney on my way to the OR, we passed by a mirror above the sink. I was shocked at my reflection. My face was completely round.

"Why didn't any of you tell me that I look like Petunia Pig? What has happened to me?"

Dr. Volpe chuckled as he replied. "You can't pump a body with 18 units of blood, seven units of platelets, and numerous bags of other i.v. liquids during a 36-hour period without getting some fluid retention. Believe me, you'll need all of that during your surgery."

When we got to the elevator, I said goodbye to my parents. Jack gave me a special farewell kiss and wished me good luck. As the elevator door began closing, I called to Jack: "I love you. Take good care of the kids."

The operating room was alive with activity. In addition to Dr. Gregory, there were three other physicians prepared to assist.

Before the anesthesia was administered, I looked up at Dr. Gregory and his colleagues. "I have every faith and confidence that you'll find the bleeding," I began. "I want to wish you good luck!"

As the anesthesiologist's countdown started, I wondered if I would ever see the faces of my loved ones again.

Chapter Thirteen

I wasn't exactly sure where I was as the cobwebs began to clear from my head. The first things my eyes focused on were white flowers—dozens of Easter lily blossoms. It seemed that I was completely surrounded by them. My first thought was that I didn't survive the surgery.

After a few more moments of wondering whether the next apparition I might see would be St. Peter or his opposite number, I then realized where I was. I began to recognize the familiar surroundings of a hospital room. I *hadn't* died after all. But I was still unclear whether they had found the source of the bleeding, since I noticed the i.v. bottles were still attached to my arm.

I finally figured out that the lilies had been sent to me by our friends. Being very practical, they probably reasoned that the lilies would be appropriate no matter which way the surgery had gone!

"Are you finally awake, Mary?" Dr. Gregory beamed as he entered the room. "I tried to tell you the good news last night in the recovery room, but you were too drifty."

"So you found the bleeding?" I asked cautiously.

"We sure did! But it wasn't easy. It was like finding a needle in a haystack," Dr. Gregory continued, his eyes alight with enthusiasm.

"Oh, thank heaven you found it! I thought I was a goner. I know my family will be relieved."

"I told Jack the good news last night. He reacted as if a heavy weight had been removed from his shoulders."

"Where did you find it?"

"It was in the small intestine. We had to pull out the entire length of your intestinal tract and lay it on your chest. We then went through it inch by inch, using our thumbs and forefingers trying to detect the bleeding source. But we found nothing the first time through the 26 feet."

"How many times did you have to go through it?"

"I decided that even though time was running out, we had to try one more time. We got lucky about half way through on the second go around. We found a hole about the size of a pea directly over a small artery."

"Do you think my cancer has spread to that area?"

"No, we think it was caused by your chemotherapy. However, we took the precaution of removing about a foot on either side and then resectioning your gut."

Dr. Gregory methodically checked the i.v. bottles. "I think this will be your last unit of blood. We'll continue the other fluids until your system begins to function again. It may take a few days because when we stuffed everything back into your abdominal cavity, I know it wasn't the same arrangement as you had before."

"That's okay, just as long as everything is tucked in," I laughed as the tension of the last three days began to subside.

"Dr. Bach, the surgical resident, will be following you on a daily basis. Of course, I'll be checking on you periodically as well." Dr. Gregory's beeper summoned him to the operating room.

As Dr. Gregory headed for the OR, I realized that this was my third different ward at Bethesda since January.

My musing was interrupted by the arrival of a tall, thin, gray-haired lady, who introduced herself as Marion Johnson, my roommate. She explained she was admitted because of a flare-up of diverticulosis, with surgery a distinct possibility.

"I've been enjoying your beautiful Easter lilies ever since they began arriving. I tried to arrange them around your bed so you could see them."

"I'm sure glad you enjoy them," I responded, trying to mask my opinion of that particular flower.

Our horticultural discussion was cut short by the ward nurse. "You're due in X-ray in ten minutes, Mrs. Johnson."

"I'm waiting for the blood bank tech," Marion responded.

"Never mind that, he'll come back," Mrs. White countered as she approached my bed, and Marion headed for X-ray.

When we made eye contact, there was simultaneous recognition.

"Mary Walker!" she exclaimed. "I had no idea it was you when I saw the name on the chart. I understand you came through the surgery with flying colors."

Bonnie White's husband and Jack had been assigned to the same Navy station a few years earlier. While we were not close friends, we got to know them pretty well after a couple of years together.

Over time, Bonnie managed to be quite well known at the officers' club as well. Frequently, after a few drinks, she became completely uninhibited, and she turned into the floor show. Her favorite "act" required the skill of Houdini and the body of a contortionist. She would place a glass filled with Scotch and water on the dance floor. Then she stood about four feet away from the glass with her back facing it. Next, in an amazing series of acrobatic moves, she would perform a stupendous back bend so that her lips ended up touching the glass. Somehow, she then took hold of the top of the glass with her mouth and teeth and slowly raised her body upward out of the bend. As her body moved toward the vertical position, she consumed the liquid in the glass. By the time she regained an upright position, the glass was empty.

Bonnie never performed her trick at the hospital, but she and the other surgical-ward nursing staff members gave me superb care during my recuperation.

Not long after Marion left the room, a young corpsman carrying a tray came in.

"Mrs. Johnson?" he asked as he looked around the room.

"No, I'm Mary Walker."

"Oh, Mrs. Walker! You made it! We were getting so many requests for you at the blood bank. When they stopped, we all figured you'd either died or gotten fixed up. Now I can let everyone know what happened to you."

As he exited my room, looking for Marion, I thought that as happy as he was, it was only a fraction of the joy I felt at having another chance at life.

Jack and my parents were still feeling a sense of relief and gratitude over the success of my surgery as they showed up precisely at the start of visiting hours.

After a joyous round of greetings, I brought them up to date on the latest information I had.

Before Jack left that day, I asked him to do me a favor.

"Anything you ask, Mary, darlin'," came the predictable response.

"I'd like for you to find new homes for these Easter lilies. Maybe you can find someone who'll enjoy them more than me," I said in obvious understatement.

Jack took them two at a time to other deserving souls. When he had relocated the last plant, he reported that all of the new owners were delighted with their unexpected gifts. They're probably still wondering today who the nut was who gave away all those beautiful Easter lilies.

Even now, when I see that flower, I am reminded of that time when I came so close to leaving those I love so much.

Dr. Bach routinely checked my abdomen with her stethoscope several times each day, listening for bowel sounds. In the meantime, I was limited to a liquid or soft food diet.

By the third day after surgery, I began to have non-family visitors. One of the first such visitors greeted me in her distinctive way: "*Guten Tag, mein Freund!* [Good day, my friend]!"

The greeting came from Marlies Buhler, one of my best friends from Bremerhaven, Germany. She and her husband, Alex, also were stationed in Washington, D.C.

Marlies and I were about the same age, but that's where the similarity ended as far as background is concerned. While she had suffered considerable hunger and hardship during World War II, I can remember feeling deprived without a steady supply of bubble gum during the war years. She said those Movietone News sequences showing ragged waifs sifting through mounds of garbage looking for food could have been depicting her. She recalled that when the U.S. forces conquered her part of Germany, they gave the people peanut butter—all the peanut butter they could eat. Due to the unpleasant memories of those years, peanut butter is not her food of choice today.

Seeing Marlies reminded me again of our hectic first week in Bremerhaven.

Jack and I were being transferred from Puerto Rico to Bremerhaven during the late summer of 1962. Rather than ship our American car to Germany, we decided to order a new Volkswagen "Beetle" for delivery upon our arrival in Europe.

About four days after our debarkation, our new car was ready at the VW factory in Wolfsburg, about 150 miles away, a stone's throw from the East German border.

Since we were between automobiles, the only viable way to get to the factory was by train.

Marlies worked as a secretary in the Navy legal office and was one of the first German nationals we met. She assured Jack that going by train from Bremerhaven to Wolfsburg would be a piece of cake. The only slight potential hitch was that we would have to transfer trains at Hannover. To make it even easier, she wrote out on a piece of paper and gave Jack the German words we would need to make our transfer.

Because Hannover was located in the British sector of occupation following World War II, there were no American troops stationed in that part of Germany. Therefore, the general public was not exposed to many Americans.

True enough, the first leg of our journey was uneventful. The *Hauptbahnhof* [main railway station] at Hannover was typically German in character. It was essentially a huge barn with open ends. Numerous trains were coming and going on what appeared to be at least a couple of dozen different tracks.

As we alighted from our train, we approached the first official-looking person in the station, a middle-aged man in a railway uniform quite reminiscent of Germany's Nazi past.

Jack's face was cast in a smug expression as he pulled out Marlies' piece of paper and read the words with great deliberation: *"Wo ist der Zug nach Wolfsburg?* [Where is the train to Wolfsburg?]"

The official replied unhesitatingly, *"Gleis elf* [track eleven]," glanced at his watch, and moved on.

Jack and I looked at each other in disbelief. We knew how to ask the question. But Marlies hadn't prepared us to understand the response.

Jack figured out that *"Gleis"* meant "track," after seeing several direction signs using that word followed by Arabic numerals. But what number was *"elf?"* The only elf I knew anything about was small, wore a green suit, and had pointed ears.

We ran from station platform to platform trying to figure out a way to decipher the word *elf*. But nowhere did we see the name "Wolfsburg" or any other clue which could help us solve the *elf* mystery. Jack made several attempts to ask other passengers where we could catch our train. Each person queried shrugged his shoulders and gave a look of indifference.

Finally, a professorial-looking man in his fifties with a gray goatee approached us. In impeccable English he asked if he could be of help.

He chuckled as he learned of our dilemma. He told us we needed to find track eleven, and he pointed out a platform about six tracks away from where we were. He also observed that the train had just completed loading and was about ready to pull out.

We thanked our kind benefactor profusely and began a mad dash toward our train. The route to our platform was circuitous, and we had to go through several tunnels beneath the other tracks to reach our destination. As we emerged from the tunnel at *Gleis elf*, our train was already moving at a pretty good clip. Instinctively, Jack and I began running alongside, just as we had seen people do in old foreign movies. Before we ran out of platform room, Jack opened the sliding door, and we both lunged forward into the moving railway car, landing on our rear ends.

Looking around the car to get our bearings, we noticed that about 50 pairs of eyes were intently focused on us. As we scrambled into the only available seats, we suddenly realized that in our hurry to catch the train, we had inadvertently ended up in the third-class area. Judging from the appearance of the passengers, we could have been riding a train in Siberia rather than in West Germany. Passengers were seated around the entire perimeter of the car, facing each other. Some were carrying primitive suitcases and bedrolls, others had live poultry tucked under their arms, and one old gent wearing wooden shoes and *lederhosen* [leather pants] had a baby goat in tow.

An old woman seated to my right kept her eyes fixed on us for the entire journey. She was short and plump, with a round, red face, covered with warts and chafed by exposure to too many northern European winters. Her grayish-yellow hair was wrapped in a dirty babushka. From the smell which emanated from her body, it was obvious that deodorants were unknown to her.

Jack and I sat in silence for the hour and a half ride—never out of the intense scrutiny of our fellow passengers—hoping we were on the right train.

When the train finally pulled into a *Bahnhof* [railway station] clearly marked "Wolfsburg," Jack and I looked at each other in relief.

As the only Americans on the train, we were easily spotted by our Volkswagen host. He drove us to the factory where we had a short tour and lunch in the executive dining room.

After lunch we were presented with our new car, and we

The Fat Lady Hasn't Sung

drove to a nearby service station to fill our gas tank for our return trip to Bremerhaven.

As Jack paid the attendant, the young German said, *"Haben Sie eine gute Fahrt."*

Jack's German had improved to the point where he replied, *"Danke schön* [thank you]," even though neither of us were quite sure what the attendant had said to us.

As Jack got back into the car, he looked at me and smiled, "Did that guy say what I thought he said?"

"It sounded like he said 'F-A-R-T,'" I grinned, as we both broke out in laughter.

As soon as we got back to Bremerhaven we both signed up for a night course in conversational German.

We finally found out that *Fahrt* meant trip, and the young lad in Wolfsburg had wished us a good one.

Just as we had solved the *elf* mystery, we eventually figured out the *Fahrt* puzzle.

CHAPTER FOURTEEN

Ten days after my emergency surgery, I had recovered enough to go home. My recovery had been slower than normal due to my inactivity. But normal bowel sounds returned within six days, and, after that, it was just a matter of time until I could be discharged.

Dad had gone back to Minneapolis to his job after he was sure I was on the road to recovery. But his daily telephone calls kept him in touch and were always a treat for me.

It was great to be home again! In spite of Jack's busy schedule, he and Mom had kept the house tidy, if not completely dust free. (Jack is an extremely neat person, but he is willing to live with a little dust here and there when he is pushed for time.)

On the second day home, I began to experience a great deal of gastrointestinal discomfort. I kept telling Mom, mostly in jest and out of frustration, that I just had to get up and walk to get some relief. Although I wasn't serious, she panicked at the thought of me trying to walk on my impaired legs.

By the time Jack returned home from work, I was vomiting about every 30 minutes. One of the conditions of my release was that I would return to the hospital as soon as possible if anything unusual occurred. Both of us agreed that my vomiting fell into that category. So, it was back to Bethesda as soon as Jack changed clothes and got my things organized.

I was re-admitted immediately and sent directly to the surgical ward. Much to my chagrin, we discovered that the surgical resident now in charge of the ward was Dr. Bach. My past exposure to her revealed that she had a unique way of "talking down" to patients, and that caused me to react defensively when I was around her.

Dr. Bach immediately concluded that the source of my discomfort was an intestinal blockage and ordered an i.v. and X-rays which confirmed her diagnosis. She also introduced me to my first but, unfortunately, not my last naso-gastric (NG) tube. Dr. Bach inserted one end of a clear, plastic tube, slightly larger than a straw in diameter, into my nose. As the tube reached the throat area, she repeatedly asked me to swallow. After numerous attempts to gulp the plastic, it finally cleared my throat and reached my stomach. Dr. Bach hooked up the other end of the tube to a pump which began to suck out the green bile which was causing me so much agony. As much as I hate NG tubes, which always make my nose sore and my throat raw, I did get almost instantaneous relief. It is amazing that the human body produces so much gastric juice per day. And with an intestinal blockage, all that liquid has no place to go except back up the esophagus to be regurgitated.

Dr. Bach, in her own inimitable way, kept the NG tube down me for the next nine days. She rejected all other possible medical protocols in favor of her beloved tube. Sure enough, the long-awaited sounds emanating from my abdomen were detected by Dr. Bach's ubiquitous stethoscope. She declared my blockage had broken and pulled my NG tube. As a precaution, I remained hospitalized for the next three days, but I resumed a normal diet.

Late on Friday before Mother's Day, Dr. Bach once more declared me fit enough to be released from the hospital. When I got home, it was obvious that Mom was exhausted, both physically and emotionally, from the events of the past several weeks. Although she hated leaving us and said she felt like a rat deserting a sinking ship, she seemed relieved when Jack and I assured her that we would get along fine without her. The next day she boarded a plane for Minneapolis.

Jack wanted just the four of us to celebrate Mother's Day in a special way. He knew that the kids and I loved to go to Peter Pan Inn, a rustic, family-style restaurant, filled with antique furniture and art deco objects, located in rural Maryland about 50 miles from Washington, D.C.

After attending church services at the Navy Chapel at Bethesda, the four of us headed for Peter Pan Inn. It was a typically bright day in May with the radiant blue sky gleaming in sharp contrast to the emerald-green fields of the Maryland countryside.

Our dinner was superb. The Southern-style fried chicken was accompanied by an impressive array of fresh vegetables, topped off with peach cobbler for dessert. Although I'm not normally a large eater, the special nature of the day combined with my enforced austerity regarding food intake during my twelve days in the hospital resulted in my eating a large, delicious meal.

After dinner David and Amy teased and chased the peacocks which paraded around the boxwood-trimmed grounds of the inn.

We couldn't have traveled more than ten miles on our return trip to Rockville when I frantically shouted to Jack: "Pull over to the side! I feel sick!"

Jack complied immediately. Before he could come around to open my door, I had pushed it open and had lost most of my dinner. He held my head as I vomited the remainder of my meal.

As he wiped my lips with his handkerchief, his voice was troubled. "What in the world do you suppose is causing this? Surely you don't have another blockage!"

"My intestinal track is still sensitive from the surgery. It'll be okay soon. I just ate too much today," I reassured him.

"I just have this horrible feeling that the cancer might have spread," Jack continued. "They haven't been able to give you any chemotherapy since your bleeding episode. I just hope they're not waiting too long. Shouldn't we go back to Bethesda?"

"No. They'll just put another NG tube in me. I'll be okay in a couple of weeks. I'm just going to take it easier from now on with what I eat."

In addition to her company, one of the big things we missed with my mother gone was her driving me to physical therapy, which I was now attending three times a week. (I had been going to PT five days a week for the first few weeks after being released from my hip surgeries.) These sessions had been part of my ongoing rehabilitation from the beginning, with the ultimate goal of getting me on crutches and out of a wheelchair. As soon as some of the Navy wives learned of my transportation needs, they devised a rotating schedule to drive me to PT. This same group of friends also had generously provided numerous meals for Jack and the kids during my earlier hospitalization.

My efforts to consume more liquids and softer foods paid off for about ten days. But later in May I was re-admitted to Bethesda once again for severe gastrointestinal distress and vomiting. Predictably, Dr. Bach started an i.v., inserted an NG tube, and primed the pump. Once again, I got almost immediate relief.

My unplanned hospitalization coincided with a scheduled, routine follow-up appointment in orthopedics. When Dr. Slimmons found out I was on the surgical ward, he kept the appointment by coming by my hospital room. He gave me a quick examination and was pleased with the progress I had made in physical therapy. As he checked my range of motion and my other joints, he noticed me wince as he moved my left shoulder back and forth.

"Do you have pain there, Mary?" Dr. Slimmons asked as he methodically checked my joint.

"Well, yes, a little. I must have pulled something swinging on the monkey bar."

"While you're here in the hospital, I think we ought to get another bone scan on you. I'll order one as soon as you get disconnected from your NG tube."

Four days after re-admission, Dr. Bach declared me "unblocked" again and pulled the abominable tube which was fast becoming my nemesis. She wanted me to stay in the hospital for a couple more days, but I was free to move around in my wheelchair.

I wheeled myself down to the bone scan area and presented Dr. Slimmons' order to the technician. It seemed almost incredible that in about a year of complaining of pain and with a positive cancer diagnosis, this was only my second bone scan. (My first scan was made in January just before starting my radiation treatment. It revealed the cancer was confined to both my hips). But, in 1974, bone scans were rather new, and they certainly were not ordered routinely.

Bone scan procedures in those days were relatively primitive compared with the state-of-the-art techniques used today. I was injected with a radioactive dye and then had to wait for about four hours for the dye to infiltrate my system. I jokingly used to warn Jack to keep away from me during this time to avoid hazardous radiation exposure. I'm sure I could have set off a Geiger counter without too much difficulty. Once the scan began, the machine traversed my body for about an hour on one side and then another hour on the reverse side. The final result of this effort was a page-sized replica of my entire skeleton, clearly showing any so-called "hot-spots" or areas of cancer activity.

The next day Jack showed up at his usual time after work and before going home. With Mother gone, he had to depend on Hilda Ponder, Sheila Sullivan, and some of the other neighbors to watch David and Amy for a couple of hours each day after school before he could get home.

Jack had visited with me for only about five minutes when Dr. Slimmons, accompanied by Dr. Perlin, appeared at the door. Both doctors wore solemn expressions.

After greeting us, Dr. Slimmons got right to what was on his mind. "Mary, the bone scan results are back." Dr. Slimmons paused for a moment, and, having known me since January, probably expected me to throw in a question.

After a few more seconds Dr. Perlin interjected, "the cancer has metastasized to the upper end of your left humerus bone."

Jack and I looked at each other, not fully aware of the exact medical terminology Dr. Perlin had used. I finally sought clarification. "Does that mean that the cancer has spread to my left shoulder?"

"I'm afraid that's exactly what has happened," Dr. Slimmons continued. "That would account for the pain you've been having there."

Jack stood in silence, his face ashen-gray. He looked totally devastated by the news.

After another long period of silence, I finally spoke. "Well, gentlemen, what's the new game plan?"

"Due to your intestinal surgery, we haven't been able to be as aggressive with your chemotherapy as we would have liked," Dr. Perlin said, almost apologetically. "But we have to attack this new spot quickly and tenaciously."

"Are you going to use radiation or chemotherapy?" Jack asked, having somewhat regained his composure.

"Both," Dr. Perlin quickly responded. "I'm reworking your chemotherapy protocol now, and we want to start with that. Then, we'll follow up with radiation for a couple of weeks."

By prior arrangement with Dr. Bach, I busied myself the next day getting my things packed to go home. Shortly before Jack was scheduled to pick me up, Dr. Perlin arrived with a large envelope filled with papers. He seemed a bit more upbeat than he was the day before.

"I've changed your chemotherapy, and I've decided to try a new, experimental drug—with your permission, of course," Dr. Perlin began. "It's called Adriamycin, and it's from Italy. But it's so new that it hasn't been approved yet by the Food and Drug Administration."

"Does it work well on my type of cancer?"

"Early studies have shown some positive indications. As I said yesterday, I think we need to hit this new activity hard and fast. This drug may be just the thing."

"Sounds good to me. When can we start?"

"Not so fast, Mary. Because it's still experimental, we need to have you sign this consent form before we can administer it."

Dr. Perlin pulled out a blank form from his envelope and handed it to me. The form was written in typical legal jargon. The gist of it was that the United States Government, in general, and the Bethesda Naval Hospital, in particular, would be absolved from any legal responsibility if I should die from taking the drug Adriamycin.

I read the disclaimer carefully, asked a few more questions, and then signed it. Dr. Perlin said it would take a few days to have the drug shipped to Bethesda.

As I waited for Jack to come and take me home, I remembered what he had said when he first started teaching me about opera. Lots of wonderful things have come from Italy, he used to say. As I finished packing the last of my belongings, I thought how prophetic Jack would be if this new drug could arrest the spread of my disease.

Chapter Fifteen

Dr. Perlin kept me busy the week following my release even though I was technically an out-patient.

One of the first procedures he ordered was another bone marrow aspiration to determine if the cancer had spread to the blood. Once again a long needle pierced the skin and tissue and crunched through the pelvic bone to reach the marrow inside.

Dr. Perlin also ordered a white blood count to determine my readiness for the next chemotherapeutic attack.

When all the procedures were completed and the results were back, Dr. Perlin asked me to stop by his office after my PT session. The files and charts which surrounded him earlier seemed to have increased since my last visit. He looked up from his clutter as I navigated a passage with my wheelchair through his office.

"Hello, Mary. It looks like everything will be ready for us to start your new chemotherapy next Monday." Dr. Perlin continued to flip through pages of paper as he talked.

"How did my tests turn out?"

"Your bone marrow was fine. There was no evidence of

cancer spreading there. I am a bit concerned about your white blood count, however."

"Is it low?"

"It's lower than we like for it to be when we start chemotherapy. I'm sure you know that it's important to maintain good nutrition during therapy."

Of course I knew. But I never told Dr. Perlin how I was subsisting mostly on liquids and soups in order to avoid another blockage. Even Jack didn't realize the extent to which I was avoiding solid foods. It was a Catch-22 situation. If I ate too much, I might get another blockage; if I ate too little, my low white blood count could prevent me from having my needed treatments.

Dr. Perlin explained my new chemotherapy recipe. "We plan to start out with Adriamycin plus four other drugs: Nitrogen Mustard, Velban, Bleomycin, and Methyl-prednisolone. Our plan is to inject a large dose of one drug each day for five days. Then, after a two-week rest, we begin the cycle again."

"What sort of reaction might I expect?"

"All of the drugs you'll be taking have the potential to cause nausea, vomiting, constipation, mouth dryness, depression, numbness, depilation, and, of course as you know, internal bleeding."

"Did you say depilation?"

"Oh, yes, I'm sorry. That means loss of hair. Some patients have all of those reactions and more, while others have just some of them."

Jack took leave the week of June 3rd in order to be with me for my first new treatment of chemotherapy. Understandably, we were both rather apprehensive about this new beginning in view of the last disaster.

Dr. Perlin had everything in readiness as we showed up at the oncology treatment room. I took a seat in what appeared to be a modified arm chair, and Dr. Perlin began a systematic search for an available vein. After just one previous chemotherapy treatment, my peripheral veins already were in poor condition. Even before my illness, anyone drawing blood from me complained that my veins were small and tended to "roll." Finally, Dr. Perlin found a suitable vein in my forearm, and he gently forced the needle at the end of a large vial containing cranberry-colored liquid through my skin and into my blood stream. Within a couple of minutes, the container of Adriamycin was empty. (In those days, this was standard technique. Today, of course, chemotherapy drugs are given by i.v. over a much longer time period in order to minimize toxicity and adverse reactions.)

Jack quickly rolled me to our car, which he had temporarily parked just outside the clinic door, and drove straight home. By the time we got there, the first waves of nausea were starting. As soon as Jack finished helping me lie down, I told him I had to get to the bathroom immediately. I made it to the commode just in time as I spewed up my breakfast. After Jack helped me back into bed, he disappeared into the children's playroom. He returned in a few seconds carrying a pink plastic container. I recognized it immediately as a doll's bathtub we had given Amy the previous Christmas.

"Use this whenever you have to vomit. Then you don't have to worry about making it to the bathroom in time."

Thus began what would become a three-year relationship between me and that notorious "pink pan."

About fifteen minutes after my first vomiting spell, another cycle of nausea and vomiting hit me. Jack was right. The pink pan made my ordeal a little less difficult. Thank goodness he was around to empty it for me.

The same cycle continued at about fifteen to twenty-minute intervals for the next eight hours as a new wave of gut-wrenching nausea and violent vomiting hit me again and again. After the first hour or so there was nothing left in my stomach to bring up except green bile. Poor Jack felt helpless as he could only offer me words of encouragement and a wet wash cloth to soothe my brow.

When the nausea finally began to subside, and I realized I was back in the realm of the living again, Jack urged me to try to drink some liquids. Nothing he suggested—juices, water, tea—

appealed to me, even though I felt thirsty and completely dehydrated. Although I normally don't care for soft drinks, when Jack suggested several varieties, I agreed to try. He opened a Coca Cola, a 7-Up, a Dr. Pepper, and a root beer. I took a sip of the first three, but I felt signs of nausea returning. Oddly enough, when I sipped the root beer, it seemed to set well with my stomach. I slowly continued to drink the root beer until I had downed the entire twelve ounces. Much to my delight, I kept the drink down, and I began to feel better. I still ached all over from the ravages the Adriamycin was bringing to my cells. But at least the nausea and vomiting had passed.

Jack had fixed supper for the kids, and a couple of hours after they had eaten, I finally felt like eating a light meal. By bedtime, I was feeling reasonably well again.

Early the next morning we were on our way back to Bethesda to repeat the ordeal of the previous day. Although the drug was different, the result was the same: hours of nausea and uncontrollable vomiting. As the week progressed, it seemed my recovery from the nausea got a bit shorter each day, and Jack was able to give me my root beer somewhat earlier each time. We were both so relieved when Friday came at last. When I was finally recovering from the effects of my last injection of that cycle, Jack joined me in a root beer toast to celebrate being off the chemotherapy for the next two weeks. Two weeks of freedom! What a wonderful thought! What a pleasure it would be to live just a normal life again, even for two weeks, without constant nausea and aching.

Jack and I spent a quiet weekend at home since I was still quite weak. The phone rang just after Jack left for work on Monday morning. It was Dr. Perlin. He asked me to report to the radiation therapy clinic on Wednesday to begin treatments on my left shoulder.

Dr. Beatty greeted me like a long-lost friend when I returned to his domain. He wanted to know how my legs were doing, and he was delighted to hear that I was nearing the point when I could use crutches.

After our initial greetings, he took a pencil and paper and began to draw a sketch of my left shoulder. He explained that unlike the massive radiation to my legs, his new plan was a more controlled approach.

"We're going to use cobalt this time," Dr. Beatty said enthusiastically. "We'll be able to concentrate the radiation to just the head of your humerus and try not to damage much of the surrounding bone or tissue."

"How often will I have the treatments and for how long?" I inquired.

"We need to treat you daily—Monday through Friday—for about thirteen sessions."

Dr. Beatty produced his red indelible marker again and drew a rectangle on my left shoulder. After checking and admiring his newest sketch, he pushed me to the cobalt treatment room where I transferred to a reclining device resembling a dentist's chair. Dr. Beatty aimed the cobalt machine's light ray at the red target on my shoulder. After he was sure of the machine's position, he left me to the silence of the room and started the cobalt bombardment of the malignant tumor in my left shoulder. The gentle humming of the machine continued for about five minutes as I remained completely motionless.

When the treatment was over, Dr. Beatty re-entered the room and helped me back into my wheelchair. This same procedure was to be repeated a dozen more times before my body had absorbed a sufficient number of rads to kill the tumor. But after about the third session, the persistent pain in my shoulder had begun to subside.

By prior arrangement, on Saturday after I started my cobalt treatments, my niece, Melinda Gleason, arrived to spend two weeks with us. She had just completed her junior year in high school in Scottsdale, Arizona, and she was interested in becoming a nurse. She wanted to know more about the details of my different treatments, and first-hand exposure would provide her that opportunity. Since she had her driver's license, she would be able to take over the driving chores from the various Navy wives who continued to help us out. She also was good with the children, and David and Amy loved having her around.

Jack wanted to do something special for our fifteenth anniversary which was rapidly approaching, particularly since the past six months had been such a washout. Much to my surprise he had obtained tickets to two different productions of the Metropolitan Opera performing at Wolf Trap Farm Park for the Performing Arts just across the Potomac River in Virginia.

The first performance, on June 18, was Mozart's *Don Giovanni*, a long-time favorite of mine. On the next night, June 19, Puccini's last opera, *Turandot*, was given.

My first exposure to Mozart's masterpiece was the NBC television production starring Cesare Siepi during the first winter of our marriage. To this day, I can still recall Siepi's magnificent portrayal of the Don.

My next significant encounter with this opera was in April, 1963. Jack and I were living in Bremerhaven at the time, and one of Jack's long-time dreams was to attend a performance at La Scala Opera House in Milan, Italy. Several months prior to a scheduled two-week vacation in Italy, Jack wrote to La Scala requesting tickets for whatever performance was to be given on April 4. When the tickets arrived, they only showed the date of the performance, not which opera was to be given.

We drove into Milan late on April 3, after snow delays in some of the higher passes of the Alps.

At breakfast the next morning we met a professor of music on sabbatical leave from the University of Wisconsin. When we told him we had tickets to that night's La Scala performance, he gasped in excitement. "Do you realize how difficult it is to get tickets for that production? It's been sold out for weeks!"

Jack and I were stunned at what we had just heard. "No, we don't even know what opera is playing tonight," Jack said, looking embarrassed.

Before Jack could explain why we were so much in the dark, the professor excitedly revealed more. "The opera is *Don Giovanni*, starring Leontyne Price and a whole cast of superb international stars!"

The performance that night more than lived up to the professor's high expectations. If just being in that venerable, tradition-packed institution were not enough, we were treated to what may have been the definitive rendition of Mozart's work.

Going to hear the Metropolitan Opera at Wolf Trap was eventful, but not as memorable as the first time Jack took me to the "old" Metropolitan Opera House at Broadway and 39th Street.

Jack had attended numerous performances there in the mid-fifties while he was a bachelor stationed in Washington, D.C. But he wanted me to share the magnificence of that place with him. Dow Berggren, while not an opera lover, also wanted to go with us since it was an opportunity he had never had.

Since we didn't have the season's schedule, Jack wrote in December for three orchestra tickets for whichever opera was being performed on Saturday, February 27, 1960. Several weeks passed before the Met responded. When the tickets arrived, I was somewhat disappointed that they were for Richard Strauss' *Der Rosenkavalier*. At that time I had scarcely heard of the work, and even Jack knew only some of the music. He had heard it on the Metropolitan Opera radio broadcasts twice before, and although he had acquired numerous opera recordings, *Der Rosenkavalier* was not in his collection.

Dow had agreed to drive his car to New York, and early on the day of the performance he picked us up.

Jack felt compelled to teach Dow and me something about the opera we were about to attend before the curtain ascended. He has always felt that the time and effort invested in preparation for an opera paid off in rich dividends at the performance. Jack told us the story of *Der Rosenkavalier*, and then he tried to hum some of the music. At that time, I had no idea what it was Jack was humming. Of course, now I realize it was the waltz tune associated with Baron Ochs in Act II.

"Listen you two," Jack urged as Dow sped along the New Jersey Turnpike. "Listen to this tune: La da da da, da da da. . .

That's one of the main themes of this opera." Jack tried to carry the melody a few bars farther, but his general lack of familiarity with the score and Strauss' complex orchestral writing combined to make his voice taper off to a sigh.

I looked at Dow's crimson face and both of us exploded with laughter. But Jack was undeterred. He continued with his version of Baron Ochs' waltz tune all the way to New York, hoping something of musical value would rub off on us. Dow and I were sore with laughter as we pulled up at the Taft Hotel.

As we entered the Met that night, Jack pointed out the famous bust of Enrico Caruso in the congested entrance foyer. When we reached our seats in the orchestra, I was overwhelmed by the enormity of the place. The high, ornate proscenium in the front contrasted with the five concentric balcony seating levels above the orchestra floor which seemed to soar to the heavens. But the centerpiece of this whole scene was the magnificent gold curtain which hung in silent witness to all the great voices of the past and present which had graced this famous stage.

Act I was uneventful. But Jack was eagerly anticipating the presentation of the rose early in Act II. Later in the act when the orchestra began to play the waltz tune Jack had hummed earlier, Jack nudged me and whispered for me to tell Dow. When I glanced to my left, I saw Dow was sound asleep. When I gently poked my elbow into his side, he let out a snort that rivaled Baron Ochs' noisy outburst after he is slightly wounded by a sword. Having heard Dow's snore, Jack shrugged as if to say "let him sleep."

On the way back to the hotel we stopped at a corner on Broadway for roasted chestnuts. As Dow bit into the warm delicacy, he looked at Jack smugly. "You know, Jack, I never did hear that tune you were humming." Dow's tone seemed to imply that Jack had been humming from the wrong opera.

Jack looked at me and winked. "I can't imagine why, Dow! I can't imagine why."

CHAPTER SIXTEEN

"Ladies and gentlemen—please evacuate the club in an orderly fashion..." The voice on the public-address system repeated the plea as Jack and I looked at each other and our companions incredulously.

Our dinner had just arrived at the Bethesda Naval Officers' Club where we were celebrating our anniversary (albeit a couple of days late) with Dow and Debbie Berggren and Kirby and Sally Robinson. This was our first opportunity in over six months to resume some semblance of social life and to show our appreciation to our faithful friends for all the support they had given us during my illness.

As the club patrons began to evacuate, the six of us concluded that this must be the real thing, and we joined their ranks.

Jack pushed my wheelchair to the far end of the front parking lot where several other couples were standing. One gentleman in the group cupped his hands around the bowl of his pipe as he attempted to re-light it. I recognized his face immediately as he withdrew his hands.

"Dr. Slimmons! What a surprise to see you here! We're going

to have to stop meeting like this."

Dr. Slimmons chuckled as he introduced his wife and another couple. Jack introduced the Berggrens and the Robinsons.

"Has anyone heard what's going on," Jack inquired.

"I saw the manager on our way out. He said they had a call saying a bomb had been placed inside the club," Dr. Slimmons responded as he calmly puffed on his pipe.

This gave me the opening I wanted. "I'd like you to know, Dr. Slimmons, I had nothing to do with this bomb threat. But I could have been out here a lot sooner if you would let me use crutches."

Dr. Slimmons laughed. "Here we go again, Mary—same tune, second verse." I had been pestering him about using crutches for the past two weeks. He turned to look at Jack. "Is she always this persistent? How do you stand it?"

Jack's only response was a faint smile.

Dr. Slimmons sucked deeply on his pipe and looked back at me. "Okay, Mary, come in Monday and we'll take a look."

A few minutes later we received the all-clear signal to re-enter the club. The staff re-heated our steaks, and we resumed our anniversary dinner.

On Monday Melinda drove me to the orthopedic clinic. Dr. Slimmons seemed impressed with my ability to maneuver around on crutches, and he complimented me for having done my physical therapy exercises faithfully. He agreed to allow me to graduate from my wheelchair to crutches with the stern three-fold admonition—"don't fall, be careful, and watch where you're going." Dr. Slimmons cautioned me to always use the "four-point stance"—a technique I had been taught to use in PT—so that my hip joints never had to bear my full weight.

Progressing to crutches came just in time since Melinda was scheduled to return to Scottsdale on Sunday. For the first time in six months, I was able to drive again! What a joy to regain some degree of independence! I still had another five days of cobalt treatments to go, and I was slated to resume chemotherapy treatments on Monday. But at least I would be able to drive myself and not be a burden on someone else.

In order for Melinda not to spend her entire fortnight with us in drudgery, we found time to take her to the major monuments in Washington, plus Mount Vernon and a picnic along the Potomac, before she left. Armed with copious medical notes she had compiled during her visit, she boarded her plane on Sunday. David and Amy really hated to see her go since she was the only person since my illness began who had the time and energy to be a companion to them.

Monday morning came too quickly for Jack and me. While I was dreading another round of chemotherapy, Jack was very apprehensive about allowing me to go alone. I finally convinced him that I was perfectly capable of driving myself without his "mothering" me.

Since I knew the chemotherapy would make me sick, I decided to have my cobalt treatment first. Fortunately, I was still able to tolerate that procedure quite well.

As I entered the oncology treatment room, Dr. Perlin introduced me to a new doctor who had just arrived for duty and had been assigned to my case.

Dr. Lokey acknowledged our meeting with a soft accent which revealed his Southern origins. He was a handsome man of about 35 whose blue eyes were framed with horn-rimmed glasses. A dark, thin moustache adorned his upper lip.

Before administering the chemotherapy, Dr. Lokey gave me a mini-physical exam to determine my readiness for the new chemical onslaught. As was always the case, I had a finger stick to determine my white blood count. He then gently checked all my glands—in the throat, groin, and under my arms—for any swelling or abnormalities. Next, he examined my abdomen, locating such organs as the liver and spleen. He marked the skin on my stomach with his ballpoint pen to indicate the dimensions of my internal parts which he then measured and recorded to provide a benchmark for future comparisons. Dr. Lokey's gentleness of touch and thoroughness of examination were exemplary traits which I came to appreciate more and more over the next year.

When the results of the white blood count came back, Dr. Lokey was disappointed that my count was lower than desirable—a situation he attributed in part to my continuing radiation treatments. But in view of my last bone scan, he decided to proceed with the chemotherapy treatments as planned.

Once again, finding a suitable vein to inject the drug proved to be a painstaking struggle. When he finally found a potential candidate for receiving the injection, Dr. Lokey injected some saline solution to make sure the vein wouldn't collapse. He then took his large vial of Adriamycin and slowly discharged the entire contents into my bloodstream. Within seconds I could taste the bitter poison in my mouth. He immediately followed up with more saline solution to insure that the vein stayed open.

I wasted no time getting to the car and driving home. By the time I changed clothes and reached the bed, the first feelings of nausea hit me. What followed was almost a carbon copy of my experience exactly three weeks earlier. The pink pan, which I inaugurated during my previous treatment, was my constant companion for the next eight hours.

Jack arrived home early, ostensibly to check on the children, but more than likely to check on me. Unfortunately, there was nothing he or anyone else could do for me. The vomiting just had to run its course. When I finally asked Jack for a root beer, he was elated because he knew the end was in sight for today.

The rest of the week was essentially a repeat of the previous chemotherapy cycle. Each new day brought a new drug injection followed by about eight hours of vomiting. When Friday finally arrived, I had a double reason to be happy. It meant my last chemotherapy for this cycle *and* the end of my cobalt treatments!

Unlike the severe radiation burns to my legs, the cobalt treatments never burned my skin.

Other than being tired, I was feeling pretty well again when the weekend arrived. I commented to Jack that I felt lucky that so far I had avoided most of the adverse reactions Dr. Perlin had warned me about except for nausea and vomiting.

I guess I spoke too soon because when I washed my hair the next day, I was shocked to see a fur-lined sink where I had been washing. My hair was coming out in handfuls! Within days, my scalp was visible through the thinning strands. In two weeks I was almost bald.

I had resisted buying a wig up until this point, but with the latest scalp exposure, I decided to yield to Jack's pleas. In July of 1974 inexpensive, but attractive, synthetic wigs were not yet readily available in department stores. Consequently, we ended up paying quite a bit for a "real" wig from a specialty shop. However, the wigmakers and marketers must have learned that I was undergoing chemotherapy because within a few weeks the market seemed to be flooded with inexpensive, synthetic wigs that were not only attractive but stylish. I must have ended up with at least a dozen over the next couple of years.

The time for my next chemotherapy treatment inevitably arrived. However, my white blood count revealed my body still had not recovered sufficiently from my last treatment, and Dr. Lokey opted to postpone my injections for a week or so. Although I knew the drugs were my only road to survival, I couldn't help feeling elated by my short reprieve.

My cheerfulness was short-lived, however. About a week later that all-too-familiar feeling of gastrointestinal discomfort that I had experienced with previous blockages returned with a vengeance. By the time Dr. Bach re-admitted me to the surgical ward, I was vomiting every 30 minutes.

In her infinite wisdom, Dr. Bach decided to try a new technique to relieve my blockage. Instead of the conventional NG tube which I had experienced several times before, she produced a special tube which was weighted with a bulb of mercury at the end. The diameter of the bulb was only slightly smaller than my nostril. Getting that device from my nose through my throat, to my stomach was quite a struggle.

When it was finally in place, Dr. Bach dictated her instructions. "Lie on your side, Mary, and slowly feed the tube into your nose. We want the weighted end to enter your small intestine."

By now I'd just about gotten a bellyful of Dr. Bach's arrogance, literally and figuratively. "And I guess you expect this to come out the other end?" I asked sarcastically, my throat sore from swallowing the mercury bulb.

"That's exactly what I expect. The peristaltic movement of your intestinal tract should advance it all the way through and help break up your blockage."

When Jack returned a few hours later he found me in one of my rare episodes of depression. Not since the initial diagnosis of cancer in January had I felt so low. There was something about the new NG tube combined with Dr. Bach's condescending manner which triggered my feelings of despair.

Sensing my mood, Jack did his best to cheer me up. Just having him there and knowing how he had continued to stick by me made me feel better. And, physically, the nausea and vomiting had stopped as the NG tube continued to pump my stomach.

As Jack ended his visit, my roommate returned from her preoperation rounds which had occupied her most of the day. We introduced ourselves almost simultaneously.

Terri Donahue was a short, plump, boisterous woman about my age. She was scheduled for gall-bladder surgery the next day. As she talked about how long she had waited for X-rays, I noticed she spoke with a distinctive New England accent. When I asked her where she was from, I was not surprised to hear Boston.

I suppose she felt a need to reciprocate by asking me where I was from. When I replied that I was born in Iowa, she exploded with laughter.

"Iowa!" she screamed. "I can't believe anyone would admit being from Iowa! That's the most provincial place I've ever been!"

I couldn't believe what she was saying. Jack always told me he thought Iowa was the most typically American state in the union.

Terri continued. "When I ordered a gimlet, they didn't even know what it was. When I told them it was like a martini with an onion instead of an olive, they brought out the drink with a slice

The Fat Lady Hasn't Sung

of Bermuda onion in it! Can you believe it?"

As Terri continued to expound about how uncivilized the Midwest was, my mind tuned her out in favor of recalling a person who thought Iowa was paradise on earth.

After Jack and I returned to Bremerhaven from our train trip to Wolfsburg, we both enrolled in a night course in conversational German.

Our instructor, Herr Mavers, was a middle-aged German national who I thought was a dead ringer for the movie actor Peter Lorre. He belted his pants up midway between his waist and armpits and always looked quite uncomfortable.

Herr Mavers conducted the class in German, teaching us such useful phrases as "*Herr Braun hat zwölf hässliche Töchter* [Mr. Brown has twelve ugly daughters]," or "*Arme Leute haben kein Arme* [Poor people have no arms]."

One night after class he asked us for a ride to the *Hauptbahnhof* [main railway station] so he could catch the train for his home near Bremen.

During the ride to the train station, Herr Mavers asked where each of us were from in the States. When I said Iowa, his eyes lit up and his voice was animated.

"Iowa!" he exclaimed. "That's the most wonderful place I've ever been!"

"You've been to Iowa, Herr Mavers?" I asked, shocked by his statement.

"Yes, indeed, Frau Walker. I was a German prisoner of war during World War II, and we were sent to Algona, Iowa."

My mind flashed back to the early 1940's, and I vaguely remembered having seen barracks-like buildings on a farm near Algona, about 40 miles southeast of my hometown of Estherville.

"Those were the best days of my life," Herr Mavers enthused. "We had plenty of good food, and we were always treated well. You would never know we were prisoners of war."

He continued to extol the virtues of farm life in Iowa. "Our life was so healthy; we had lots of fresh air and sunshine. Sure, we had to work on the farms around there, but it was not unreasonable work. My dream is to return to Iowa some day to thank those people for treating us like humans."

Terri's continuing diatribe about Iowa brought me back to the reality of the present.

As I pushed a bit more of the NG tube up my nose, I thought it takes all kinds.

CHAPTER SEVENTEEN

By depression from having yet another intestinal blockage, combined with Dr. Bach's unorthodox treatment, was short-lived.

Although by nature I am not easily depressed, my sweet husband helped me regain my normal equilibrium by his daily visits and cheery countenance. Once again, Jack was alone, trying to look after the children and the house, plus keeping up with the demands of his job. In spite of the pressures on him, he always found a way to cheer me up.

My friend, Judy, also brightened up my stay with a visit. She apologized for not having come sooner, but she explained that she had spent the last few days in an encounter group session.

"Oh, Mary, I was locked up for an entire weekend with a bunch of weirdos."

"How did you get into that situation?"

"Would you believe it was mandatory for my job? We had to touch and hug and listen to everyone's problems. I even had to make up some so I could fit in."

"Was it just your office?"

"No, I didn't even know those people. I was so embarrassed." We both laughed until our sides ached as Judy continued to relate her touchie-feelie experience, including detailed descriptions of some of the more bizarre characters and situations.

"In order for me to regain my sanity, Mary, I did my born-to-shop thing. I saw this blouse and thought of you."

Inside a fancy-wrapped package was one of the most beautiful white silk blouses I had ever seen.

About six days after Dr. Bach inserted her mercury-weighted NG tube, she showed up in my room looking flustered. "What have you been doing?" she demanded.

"Just what you told me to do," I responded defensively. "I've been pushing this tube down."

"The X-rays show the end of the tube is *still* in your stomach! It has never entered your intestines. It's been winding around in a circle."

"Maybe the trap door won't open," I said sarcastically as she cut me short.

"We'll have to pull the tube now! If it has formed a knot, we're in serious trouble."

"What would that involve?" I asked, still puzzled by her frantic appearance.

"We would have to remove it surgically."

Dr. Bach slowly began pulling the tube hand over hand, like a sailor hoisting an anchor, stopping periodically when the resistance became more taut. When I felt the mercury tip forcing its way up my throat and out my nose, we both heaved a sigh of relief.

Dr. Bach's countenance changed from being frantic to her normal arrogance. "The good news is the blockage is breaking up. The rest must have been good for your system. We'll keep you here a few more days to monitor your progress."

Other than having a sore throat and nose, I was feeling pretty well again after my ordeal with the tube.

A couple of days later, Dr. Lokey appeared with my chart under his arm.

"Mary, your white blood count is finally back to an acceptable level. I feel like we can't wait any longer to start your next treatment cycle. It'll soon be two weeks late."

I had been expecting to hear those words, although just having gotten relief from my intestinal discomfort, I dreaded to start a new round of vomiting and nausea. But I nodded my acquiescence anyhow.

"Good. Then I'll arrange to have you brought down to the clinic later this morning so we can get started."

Once again, Dr. Lokey was extremely thorough in all of his preparations prior to injecting the Adriamycin. As he emptied the oversized syringe, I remember thinking that I didn't have far to go before the nausea hit.

But hit it did shortly after I got back to my room. Instead of my trusty pink pan, this time a government-issued embicin basin shared my ordeal. Several hours later, as the nausea began to wear off, Jack was there with a root beer to help sooth my churning stomach.

The next morning Dr. Bach signed my release papers, and I checked out of the surgical ward one more time. Before I could go home, however, I needed to get my second chemotherapy injection in the current series.

By now my chemotherapy routine had evolved into an all-too-predictable nightmare of nausea and vomiting, followed by bone-wracking body aches and a tired, drained feeling.

My depilation, as Dr. Perlin euphemistically continued to refer to my hair loss, by now was almost complete. Not only had I lost most of the hair from my scalp, except for a thin fringe around the sides, I was rapidly losing my eyebrows and even my eyelashes.

On my first night home, after looking in the mirror, I remarked that my head was so bald that I could be on the receiving end of Minnesota Fats' pool cue.

I finished up my chemotherapy cycle just in time for Mom's and Dad's visit. Dad had retired recently after spending most of his life in the grocery and produce business, and they were moving from Minneapolis to Mesa, Arizona, to start a new life in a less hostile climate. They traveled a rather circuitous route to their Promised Land via Rockville to spend several weeks with us.

Their visit was a godsend. Not only were they a tremendous help around the house and with David and Amy, but they also brought a stabilizing sense of family unity which had been missing since my illness began.

Several days after their arrival, all of us (except Jack who was working) went shopping for back-to-school clothes and supplies for the children. David and Amy had a good time picking out new lunch boxes. And Mom and I enjoyed helping the kids select new clothes.

We decided to have lunch at a restaurant in the shopping center. While everyone ordered chili dogs, I opted for a vanilla shake.

Dad wanted me to join him in his gastronomic treat. "Why don't you have one of these, Honey?" Dad asked as he displayed his hot dog with both hands. "They're really good."

"No, thanks, Dad. I'll just let sleeping dogs lie," I grinned. "I'm not too hungry. After I get home I'll have some bouillon."

I had been consuming primarily liquids all summer in order to avoid another blockage. And since my last bout with the NG tube, I had been taking liquids almost exclusively.

By the time we arrived home, I had to race on my crutches to get to the bathroom before I lost my milk shake. I was beginning to feel like Old Faithful because during the spring and summer I believe I spewed up more food than I had consumed.

I couldn't believe I had another blockage after following my liquid diet for the past few weeks. But at Mom's and Dad's urgings, I called Dr. Lokey who told me to come to his office.

As soon as I arrived, Dr. Lokey ordered a blood count. When the results returned, he looked grim.

"*What* have you been eating?"

Before I could respond, he answered his own question. "Precious little, according to your blood!"

I tried to explain how I had been on a fluid diet to avoid another blockage.

Dr. Lokey shook his head. "You can't come back from chemotherapy treatments without proper nutrition, Mary." His expression was still somber. "I'm going to admit you again until we get to the bottom of this problem."

"Do you think the cancer has spread to my intestinal tract?"

"I don't know. Anything is possible with this disease."

As I approached the surgical ward desk, I spied Dr. Bach perched there like a vulture. Oh, No! I thought. Another round with the Wicked Witch of the West. Ours was truly a love-hate relationship. Professionally, she was competent; but her interpersonal relationships left much to be desired.

"I see you're back again, Mrs. Walker. Maybe the fourth time will be the charm."

"I sure hope so." I smiled faintly.

"This time I won't be following your case. This is my last day on the ward."

As Dr. Bach told me her news, I felt like jumping up and singing the *Hallelujah Chorus*.

"When you get settled in your room, I'll bring by my relief to meet you."

A few minutes later, Dr. Bach, accompanied by a handsome man, entered the room. Dr. Bach introduced Dr. Kingsley and began briefing him on my background. As the doctors talked, his Southern accent was in sharp contrast to Dr. Bach's basic Bronx. Dr. Kingsley was about Jack's age and size. I thought if he hadn't made it as a doctor, he could have tried the movies with his matinee-idol good looks.

When Dr. Bach left the room, Dr. Kingsley turned to me and smiled.

"I'm sorry, Mrs. Walker, but we're going to have to use the NG tube again until you get stabilized. I wish there was some other way." His empathy for patients was readily apparent. "After you get some relief, I'm going to order a couple of barium tests to see if we can figure out what's causing your problem."

As Dr. Kingsley deftly inserted a regular NG tube, I thought either I was getting used to this procedure or he had an unusually gentle touch. Within minutes, the pump was removing the gastric juices causing my discomfort, and I began to feel better.

I knew immediately that I was going to like Dr. Kingsley. Somewhere along the way, I seem to have developed a penchant for Southern men. First and foremost there was Jack, although he claims to be a Southwesterner. More recently, Dr. Lokey appears to be an ideal oncologist. And now, Dr. Kingsley seems determined to solve my current problem. All three men display the same paradoxical characteristic of being at once strong but gentle.

In a few days my system returned to normal, and Dr. Kingsley pulled the NG tube and ordered an upper and lower gastrointestinal series. During rounds the next day, he stayed on to discuss my options.

"Mary, the barium tests were unremarkable—that is, they failed to reveal the exact reason for your blockages."

"Do you have any idea what's causing them?"

"It's really hard to say. It could be any number of things. Of course, we can't discount your disease."

"What options do I have?"

"We could continue treating you conservatively in the hope that your symptoms will eventually disappear. Or, we could do exploratory surgery."

As much as I dreaded hearing that word again, I wanted to get off the NG tube treadmill.

"What do you recommend, Dr. Kingsley?"

"Of course, I'm a surgeon, and I subscribe to the old cliché 'to cut is to cure.' But I'll do whatever you want me to do."

"I'm tired of marching in place, so cut away."

"Fine. I'll put you on the schedule for day after tomorrow."

The next day Dr. Kingsley looked frustrated as he informed me that the operating rooms had become contaminated and were closed for surgeries until sterile conditions could be restored.

"You have the option of going to Walter Reed for the surgery or marking time here until our OR is ready."

"Would you be doing the surgery there?"

"They might let me swab the decks, but no cutting," he laughed.

"Guess I'll just keep on marching here."

I never did find out what caused the contamination, but a week later I was wheeled into the OR with all systems go.

When I returned from the recovery room, Jack was waiting as usual.

"Have you heard anything from Dr. Kingsley?" Jack asked anxiously as he kissed me.

"Not really. He said he'd be by shortly."

I hardly finished my reply when Dr. Kingsley appeared, still in his scrubs.

"Well, we've solved the mystery," he smiled. "You were filled with adhesions from your last surgery. They had your intestines in knots."

"Was there any sign of malignancy?" Jack inquired nervously.

"No, everything appeared to be normal. Of course we'll have to wait for the pathology report."

Jack looked visibly relieved.

"What caused the adhesions, Dr. Kingsley?" I asked.

"Adhesions are usually a by-product of surgery," Dr. Kingsley explained in a professorial tone. "But normally they are broken up by walking and moving around. Since you couldn't walk, they really grabbed hold of you. Now that you're on crutches, hopefully they won't return."

"Does this mean I can eat real food again?"

"You bet. Did you have something special in mind?"

"It's been ages since I've had popcorn, and popcorn is my favorite snack."

Dr. Kingsley laughed, "I thought you'd want steak. However, the more fiber the better. That's what keeps things moving along."

Chapter Eighteen

"We don't have popcorn, but we do have corn on the cob," the dietician boasted as she lifted the cover from my food tray. "Dr. Kingsley told us about your fondness for popcorn, and you've been cleared to eat anything now, Mrs. Walker."

I couldn't believe that for the first time in months I now could eat "real" food without fearing a blockage. My transition to a normal diet signaled that my hospital stay was about to end. Medically, my recovery was uneventful. I was able to get up on my crutches the first day after surgery, and the vertical gash on my abdomen, which extended from above my navel to my pubic bone, was healing nicely.

Five days after my surgery, Dr. Kingsley released me from the hospital with no diet stipulations. One of the first things I did when I got home was to dispose of all the now-unnecessary bouillon cubes I had been subsisting on for the past several weeks.

Dr. Lokey had maintained close liaison with the surgical staff since my admission and reluctantly had agreed to postpone my next round of chemotherapy until the healing process was further along. But twelve days after my release, he started the injections again. Whatever fond hope I might have had that clearing away the adhesions would diminish the nausea and vomiting were dashed 30 minutes after my Adriamycin dose.

The five-day chemotherapeutic course pretty much followed the pattern I had come to expect. This time, however, I had to hold a pillow over my abdomen to help ease the pressure on my incision as I violently retched. Also, Mom and Dad were there to help me bounce back from the depths of my indisposition.

After I recovered from the current chemotherapy, other than being on crutches, the remainder of my parents' visit was almost normal. I was able to eat anything I wanted without the constant fear of vomiting. We even went shopping and occasionally met Jack for lunch at one of our favorite restaurants.

Several days before my thirty-eighth birthday, I returned to the orthopedic clinic for a routine follow-up. Dr. Slimmons greeted me effusively and inquired about my recent surgery. He lit up his pipe as he displayed my latest X-rays on his viewer.

"I've been looking at your most recent X-rays, Mary, and they've caused me to rethink our current management of your case."

Anxiety spread over my body as I waited for another shoe of adversity to drop.

Dr. Slimmons drew deeply on his pipe as he continued to examine my femur bones on the X-ray images. "Your birthday's on the twenty-fourth, isn't it?"

My mouth was too dry to respond. But I nodded affirmatively.

He continued to look at my X-rays. "Well, I've decided to give you a birthday present. You're going to walk out of here today on a cane!"

Dual emotions of relief and elation erased my anxiety. A cane! I couldn't have asked for a better birthday present. I was slowly but surely getting back to normalcy.

After a technician measured and cut the cane to my size, Dr. Slimmons cautioned me to always use it with my right hand to support my weaker left hip.

On my actual birthday, Jack took us all out to dinner at one of Washington's fanciest restaurants. For the first time in nine months, I could *walk* in unassisted except for my cane. I was beginning to feel more and more that I was rejoining the human race.

Mom and Dad resumed their much-delayed odyssey to Arizona the day after my birthday, departing with mixed emotions. They hated to leave us in my uncertain condition. But they were anxious to start the retirement they had waited for and planned so long.

Inexorably, my next chemotherapy cycle rolled around again. But due to a low white blood count, Dr. Lokey postponed it for a week.

When my treatment did start, I experienced about the same reaction from the first three drugs I had come to expect from past injections—almost instantaneous nausea followed by hours of vomiting.

After the Bleomycin injection on the fourth day, however, something different happened. My initial reaction to the drug was the usual nausea. But by mid-afternoon I began to experience the most severe itching on my back I had ever felt. Since my hands couldn't reach all the affected areas, I was happy when Amy got home from school so she could help scratch the areas I couldn't reach. But her little hands weren't up to the task.

"Amy, honey, go get your hair brush," I pleaded in desperation.

"Oh, Mom, I don't want my hair brushed now. I want to go outside and play."

"It's not for that. Please, just go get it."

When Amy suspiciously handed me the brush, I told her to use it to scratch my back.

"Oh what a relief it is!" I sighed, as Amy moved the bristles back and forth over my itching back.

After a few minutes of the boring job, Amy begged to be relieved. But when Jack got home, I enlisted him for the brush duty.

The next morning when I went in for my last shot, I told Dr. Lokey about the bizarre incident. He was shocked when he examined my back.

"*What* have you been scratching your back with?" he asked as he saw the red whelps which extended from my neck to my waist.

"I was so desperate from the itching we used a hair brush."

Dr. Lokey shook his head in disbelief. "I want to check this next week. Try not to scratch."

By the weekend the itching had stopped, but I had developed a strange, streaky, hyperpigmentation over my back and shoulders.

When I saw Dr. Lokey on Tuesday, he was still amazed at my reaction to the Bleomycin.

"I've read in the literature about patients having cutaneous toxicity, but I've never seen it first hand. I'd like to get some pictures of this."

At the hospital photo lab the photographer instructed me to strip from the waist up. He then positioned me in front of the camera.

"I hope my husband doesn't see these photos in *Playboy*," I quipped.

"That depends on how good they are when we get them developed," he kidded as he snapped several different poses.

Life for us was fairly normal for the next few weeks. For Halloween, David dressed as a tiger, Amy went as Snow White, and I accompanied them as Quasimodo, which suited my strange gait.

During this time I began to feel a new pain in my right rib cage. I dismissed it, however, as a muscle strain caused by using the cane.

When the time came for my next chemotherapy treatment, Dr. Lokey was unhappy with my white blood count.

"Mary, your count is dangerously low. You're highly susceptible to any infection or disease. For your protection, I'm going to have to admit you."

"Oh, no, not again! I could take care of myself at home,"

I begged.

"Perhaps so. But we need to insure sterile conditions to avoid any more delays in your treatments."

For the first time since my illness, I was admitted to the oncology ward. I was placed in isolation which required staff and visitors to wear masks, gloves, and sterile gowns. For an entire week, I lived like a hermit. I felt like Leonora in *La Forza del Destino*. In addition to daily blood counts, Dr. Lokey ordered a new bone scan.

On the day of my discharge, Dr. Lokey showed up with a grave look.

"Mary, the bone scan report was not good. You have several new hot spots."

That all-too-familiar feeling associated with adverse medical news swept my body again. His voice seemed to be resonating from the depths of a well.

"You have new lesions on your right lower rib cage, upper lumbar spine, lower thoracic spine, sternum, and skull."

My heart sank as he tallied up the new tumors. I now knew the reason for the pain in my right ribs. "It's spreading like wildfire even after all the chemo I've had. I can't understand it."

"We had to reduce your dosage several times because your white count didn't recover fast enough," Dr. Lokey explained.

"Why am I having so much difficulty with my white count?"

"First of all, you're a small person. And, secondly you've had massive radiation to both femurs, which are the largest marrow-producing bones in your body. Of course, you've also had cobalt on your shoulder, all of which only adds to the problem."

"Is there any way we can stop the spreading?"

"Dr. Perlin and I have discussed this at length. We've decided we have to take a more aggressive approach."

"Well, what's the master plan?"

"We're going to completely change your regimen. First of all, we have to stop the Bleomycin. You've reached the toxicity level with that. We still feel that Adriamycin is the drug that could eventually turn your case around. So we're going with higher doses of that along with two other drugs—Vincristine and Procarbazine."

I decided not to tell Jack about the latest scan until we got home and put the children to bed.

After dinner, as we sipped coffee, I got up enough nerve to tell Jack about the new hot spots. As I spoke, I could actually see the color disappear from his face. He was completely heartbroken. For the past several months he had been a pillar of strength and optimism. But now it seemed his whole world was shattered. The dam that had held back his tears and emotions and had sustained him since January was now ruptured, and all his grief poured forth like a raging torrent. We both wept uncontrollably as we held each other, more aware now than ever before that events beyond our control could end our undying love.

After a long silence, I was the first to speak.

"Jack, darling, we can't go on living this way. I've been stalked by death for almost a year now. We can't worry about every scan or every ache and pain. We've got to make each day count to the fullest. Let's try to keep our life as normal as possible."

"But you've suffered the worst kind of agony and vomited your guts out. And for what? Only to have that damn stuff spread all over your body," he sobbed.

"I'm not going to be licked by this, Jack! I'm going to fight this disease tooth and nail. If it finally claims me at the end, I'll have gone down fighting all the way."

My positive attitude seemed to help Jack regain his composure. "What are the doctors planning to do?" he asked, with dejection still in his voice.

"They've cooked up a new recipe for me, and I start it next week."

As I filled Jack in on the details of my upcoming treatment, both of us were now beginning to accept the reality of the situation we faced.

When we were getting ready for bed, I broached a new subject I'd been thinking about for some time. "Honey, how would you feel about all of us making a trip to Arizona and Texas over Christmas?"

"I don't know if it will be possible for you to be away that long. Why don't you check with the doctors at your next appointments."

"I really would like to make that trip, Jack. It might be my last opportunity to spend the holidays with our families."

The new chemotherapy course made me just as sick as the previous one, except it lasted three days instead of five and was administered every 28 days.

Dr. Lokey was pleased with our tentative plans for Christmas and agreed to work my treatments around our schedule. He also informed me they planned to start cobalt on my rib lesion in January.

During my next orthopedic checkup, Dr. Slimmons was satisfied with the healing process in my legs. However, he was very concerned about the cancer's spread to other bone areas. He also supported our proposed trip. He even gave me an early Christmas gift by allowing me to walk without a cane. However, as a precaution, he urged me to use the cane in public places.

When I told Jack about both doctors' supportive attitude regarding our trip, he readily agreed to make the travel arrangements.

Jack also had been thinking about a decision which was weighing on his mind. "Mary, I've just about decided to put in my retirement papers."

Although I knew Jack would leave the Navy one day, his statement caught me by surprise. "But I thought you wanted to wait for the next selection board to meet," I countered.

"That really doesn't matter to me anymore. If I get promoted, I have to be transferred. And there's no way I'd ever leave you in this condition."

As soon as Jack's request for two week's leave was approved, he purchased our airline tickets. The four of us were scheduled to fly from Washington to Phoenix to San Antonio and return.

He had a big smile on his face when he handed me the

tickets for safekeeping. "Merry Christmas, Mary, Darlin'! This trip is costing us a few bucks. But it's worth it."

Throughout our married life, Jack and I had always saved for the future. But as I looked over the tickets and saw how costly the trip would be for us, I thought *now* is the future.

Chapter Nineteen

I'm not sure who was more excited—David and Amy or me—as we boarded the plane at Dulles International Airport.

Our children hadn't been on a plane since we left Guam four years earlier when they were too young to know much about flying. And Jack had given me this trip because of my intense desire to see both sets of parents for what may be the last time.

Since we were traveling with small children, we boarded the aircraft before the general public, and we were seated in the first row.

The flight attendants showered David and Amy with attention, giving them everything from flight wing pins to special drinks. One attendant in particular stood out because she talked to the children every time she passed our row. She appeared to be of Japanese descent with a vivacious personality and a mercury-quick smile. She reminded Jack and me of another Japanese girl we met on a trip we took to Japan several years earlier.

About halfway through Jack's tour on Guam, he and I decided to take advantage of a free rest-and-recreation flight to Japan on an Air Force cargo plane. Another Navy couple, whose three children we had kept when they took a similar trip, agreed to look after David and Amy for the week we would be gone. (We had never left the children for an extended period before—even for overnight—so we were departing with more than normal apprehensiveness.)

As we boarded the World War II vintage airplane, I couldn't believe that in October, 1969, people were still flying around in planes which required passengers to walk "uphill" from the entrance door near the rear to the seating area up front. We sat down on canvas "bucket" seats and strapped ourselves in with oil-stained safety belts. Typically, we had to board about 45 minutes before take-off. By the time the engines popped and sputtered and started the two propellers turning, Jack was soaking wet with perspiration from the high humidity and 90-degree heat.

The flight north was uneventful, although slow by jet aircraft standards. We stopped briefly in Okinawa to refuel and stretch.

When our plane broke through a fleecy cloud escarpment about six hours after starting our trip, we could see the sand-trimmed Japanese coastline bordering the royal blue of the Pacific Ocean. As we began our descent and approached the Tokyo metroplex, the buildings, streets, and cars below all looked as congested as an ant hill.

We landed with a resounding screech of tire rubber making contact with concrete at Yokota Air Force Base in the outskirts of Tokyo and boarded a taxi for downtown.

We traveled for several miles along a multi-laned boulevard with unsynchronized traffic lights. Between red lights, our driver reached speeds of 60 or 70 miles an hour. And even though all three of us could see a stop light just changing from green to red two blocks up ahead, our driver wove in and out of traffic at top speed (like a Kamikazi pilot) zeroing in on his target—the shortest lane of cars backed up at the light.

Our destination was the Sanno Hotel, an American joint services officers' open mess and transient billeting facility, in downtown Tokyo—a long stone's throw from the Imperial Palace.

True to form, there had been a miscommunication about the intended dates of our visit. We had reservations all right—they just didn't start until the third day of our visit. We thought we could live with that since we had seen several American-style, high rise hotels nearby. The desk clerk pierced our fantasy bubble quickly, however, when he informed us that *all* the hotels in Tokyo were completely booked. If we were going to stay in the city for the next two nights, it would have to be at a *ryokan* [inn].

The clerk scratched in Japanese calligraphy the name and address of the *ryokan* he had called for us. We showed the paper scrap to a saner-looking taxi driver, and after winding through some narrow, tree-lined streets, we arrived at our lodgings in less than ten minutes.

Our *ryoken* was nestled in a lush, tree-covered sanctuary which somehow seemed to have been bypassed by the bustling city—an island of quietude in an ocean of noise and traffic.

We walked through a quaint Japanese garden—complete with stone lanterns and miniature trees—to get to the front entrance. Our *ryoken* resembled an enlarged version of a traditional Japanese home. In the entrance area, rows of bins (reminiscent of large post office boxes without fronts) covered two walls. Instinctively, Jack knew we were supposed to take off our street shoes and trade them for the slippers neatly lined up in each box.

A smiling, older woman, clad in traditional Japanese garb, greeted us at the front desk with a deep bow and a greeting: "Kon'nichiwa. *Irasshai mase?* [Good afternoon. May I help you]?"

Jack and I gave shallow return bows to our hostess. Then Jack told her our names. A look of understanding spread over her face as she nodded and produced a registration card. After we completed the form, she rang a bell which summoned a younger assistant. A pretty young girl in her late teens or early twenties, wearing a red-flowered kimono, emerged from a back room. She smiled quickly and bowed deeply.

"Me Yoko. I take you to room," she said in pidgin English. "You follow me."

We followed her up a narrow stairwell to the second floor where she opened our door, proudly showed us our lodgings, and then quickly disappeared.

Our room reminded me of a set from Puccini's Madama Butterfly, except in miniature. The "living" space consisted of an area approximately eight feet square, in the center of which was the room's only furniture—a low table, surrounded by four zabuton cushions. The "bedroom" adjoined the living area and was even smaller in size, separated by rice paper-paneled sliding doors. Our "bed" was a tatami mat on the floor, not long enough to accommodate Jack's feet. The bath was a mere cubicle containing a small sink with running water and a Japanese toilet—a hole in the floor which flushed but no seat to sit on. Jack quickly noted there was no shower for bathing.

By the time we had finished touring our room, Yoko returned carrying a tea tray. As we sat on the floor with our legs crossed, she ceremoniously poured each of us tea, accompanied by a Japanese wafer. She beamed as we sipped our tea and indicated our approval.

In our cramped quarters with our undersized cups, I felt like we were "playing house."

As Yoko was about to leave, Jack asked her about a subject I'm sure he'd been thinking about since his steam bath on the Guam Tarmac.

"Where we take bath?"

I laughed to myself as I noted Jack had reverted to an old habit of speaking English at the same level of the foreigner whose language he couldn't speak.

"Oh, we have nice bath downstairs. I bring you kimono," Yoko replied as she disappeared again.

Before we had finished our tea, Yoko returned with two kimonos. She instructed us to change to the garments and come downstairs when we were ready to bathe.

Twenty minutes later, we reported to the desk downstairs. Yoko and her older companion were together as we approached. When the Japanese women saw us, they both began giggling, covering their mouths with their hands to hide their actions.

Finally Yoko revealed the source of their amusement. "Papa san wear obi wrong," she chuckled as she began to untie the sash around Jack's waist. "Obi always tie in back." Jack had tied his belt in front like a bath robe. She quickly remedied the *faux pas*.

Yoko led us to a door at the end of the hall. We entered a large room containing what looked like a small swimming pool, about 20 feet square, with clouds of steam levitating from the heated water.

Since Jack and I had been to Europ, we were expecting a public bath where one guest at a time uses the facilities. But *not* a community bath!

Yoko reassured us that our bath would be quite private since it was mid-afternoon, and Japanese people usually bathe later in the day. She also instructed us on the points of etiquette involved in such a time-honored procedure. The bather sits on a low bench, pours a bucket or two of hot water over himself, soaps up, rinses off with another bucket of water, and *then* gets into the steaming pool to soak.

Our bodies were just getting used to the hot water when we heard animated male voices speaking Japanese. When we turned to discover the source of the distraction, much to my embarrassment we saw a quartet of Japanese men, clad in kimonos, entering the room. I slouched down in the water until only my head was visible above the steam.

I don't believe our unwelcome guests saw us at first through the thick clouds of vapor as they quickly disrobed and began pouring buckets of water over each other. After several minutes of soaping and rinsing, the thinnest member of the foursome finally noticed us in the far corner of the pool.

"*Gomen nasai. Sumi masen* [Excuse me. I am sorry]," he smiled as he bowed deeply to us. By now his three corpulent companions were aware of our presence as well as they faced us in their altogether and bowed in unison. Jack nodded his head and forced a thin smile. I was so far down in the water that if I had even bent my head slightly, my face would have been under water.

The bathers continued cavorting through the preliminary part of their bath ritual. By the time they finally got ready to go in the water, Jack and I felt like we were already cooked.

After the last member of the group eased himself into the hot water, Jack whispered: "Let's get out of here—now!"

"Not with those men in here. Let's wait until they leave," I countered as I sunk deeper into my watery protective blanket.

"Oh, come on, Mary! They're not going to pay any attention to you. I can't take any more of this heat. I'm getting out."

Jack hoisted his pink body out of the water and began drying off, motioning for me to join him.

Our Japanese associates were now really getting into the swim of things. They swam and splashed water as they played some sort of tag game. And one of the portly gentlemen floated on his back—his distended belly rising above the water's surface like a whale's back. After about 20 minutes, they finally tired of their bath, got out of the water, put on their kimonos, bowed to us, and left the room.

This was my signal to escape from my self-imposed imprisonment. My shriveled skin was ruby red as Jack helped me out and wrapped a towel around me.

As I put on my kimono, I remarked to Jack that I felt like a raisin in the Land of the Rising Sun.

The remainder of our time in Japan went fast as we toured and shopped. We saw every shrine, temple, pavilion, and historical edifice we could manage in Tokyo, Nikko, Nara, and Kyoto. In addition to shopping for our family, I bought a $250 camera for one of the medical corpsmen on Guam who had paid me in advance.

The first leg of our return flight to Guam on the same plane we had arrived on was routine, arriving in Okinawa just before sunset.

When we took off for Guam, the last rays of a brilliant sunset streaked across the darkened sky. We quickly cleared the runway, and, in short order, we were heading south over the Pacific

Ocean. We were still climbing when I noticed smoke coming up from under the door separating the cockpit from the passenger space.

Suddenly the cockpit door flew open, and the flight engineer—with panic written across his face—rushed out to the emergency exit above the right wing. He kicked out the right window and then repeated his stomp on the left side.

Fortunately, we had not attained our flight altitude, so there was no sudden decompression. But the deafening sound of the motors permeated the open-windowed interior.

By now black clouds of smoke were billowing from the cockpit into the cabin area. From the distinctive odor of the fumes, there was no doubt that we had an electrical fire.

Seconds after kicking out the windows, the flight engineer rushed back to the cockpit with a fire extinguisher and began spraying the bank of instruments which were producing the smoke.

Neither Jack nor I said a word to each other as our eyes made contact, and our hands joined. It wasn't necessary. Both of us thought that our time had come. We felt certain that the fire probably immobilized the controls or destroyed the hydraulic system, and that a best case scenario would be a crash landing at sea.

A thousand thoughts rushed through my mind as Jack and I held each other and gasped for fresh air. What would happen to David and Amy? How would our parents take the news? I thought about the corpsman on Guam who would not get the camera he'd paid for. And, as ridiculous as it now seems, I thought how different the cold waters of the Pacific Ocean would feel compared to the steamy warmth of our community bath at the *ryokan*.

My reverie was interrupted by the feel of our aircraft banking to the left. Perhaps not *all* the controls were incinerated! Now we were beginning to descend. Could we return to the runway? Would the landing gear work? There was no intercom system, and, with the sound of two propeller-driven engines roaring through the open windows, any attempt to keep the passengers informed of their fate was impossible.

My imagination continued to run on full throttle as the smoke began clearing from the passenger area. Surprisingly, throughout the whole emergency, all the passengers remained calm. No one screamed or went into hysterics. Jack and I continued to hold each other in the realization that there was absolutely nothing we could do except pray to prevent a tragedy, and if it did come, at least we would die together.

After what seemed like an eternity, we heard the wonderful sound of our landing gear being lowered. Maybe we were going to make it after all! Through the right window we caught a glimpse of the runway lights up ahead. Somehow our crew had maneuvered the wounded bird back over land with the potential for a safe landing. Sure enough, a few minutes later, the wheels gently made contact with the runway, as the passengers erupted with cheers and applause. We had made it safely by the grace of God and the skill of the crew!

We contacted our friends on Guam, explained our delay, and retired to the BOQ to spend an unexpected night on Okinawa.

When we returned to the air terminal the next day, we expected to see either a commercial plane or a substitute military aircraft. Instead, we were asked to tempt fate and reboard our ill-starred venerable plane again. In frustration, Jack checked the commercial airline schedules only to discover that the lone flight to Guam that week was four days later. The flight crew told us that maintenance personnel had worked all night to repair the damage and assured us the plane was completely airworthy once again.

Stupid or not, we boarded the plane for the last leg home and arrived uneventfully but happy.

Next day when I gave the elated corpsman his new camera, he asked how our trip had been.

"Exciting," I replied in understatement. "Almost *too* exciting."

Chapter Twenty

"Please fasten your seat belts and extinguish all smoking materials. We are ready for our final approach to Phoenix."

The sound of the flight attendant's voice announcing our imminent arrival aroused me from my ruminations of our trip to Japan.

Our plane made a picture-perfect landing and quickly taxied to our arrival gate where my beaming parents waited. Even though we had seen them just three months earlier, they greeted us as though we hadn't seen them in three years.

I don't think Dad, in particular, ever got over my having cancer. In fact, he found it difficult to even utter the word. Somehow, to him, it was just unacceptable for his "baby" to have a life-threatening disease. If he said it once, he said a hundred times that he wished it had been he who had come down with the illness instead of me.

By now my parents were settled comfortably in Mesa, one of the many burgeoning cities comprising the Phoenix metroplex. They had leased a comfortable one-bedroom townhouse in a lovely retirement community. But in order to afford us more privacy and to give our kids a chance to swim, Dad had reserved space for us at a nearby motel, complete with a heated swimming pool.

David and Amy hadn't been swimming since our Rockville pool closed when school started, so they were ecstatic about our accommodations. Even though the Arizona nights were quite cool, the bright sunshine combined with the heated water made swimming in December bearable. If the cold bothered them, our kids never dropped a hint of any discomfort. Instead, they wanted to swim almost every waking moment.

On Christmas eve the weather began to change. A low-pressure system moved in, replacing the sunny skies with a rainy-looking cloud cover. A cold north wind pushed out the warmer air, and it felt like we were back in Maryland.

For Christmas, we had a big get-together with my sister and her family, my parents, and the four of us. With the change in the weather, our Arizona Christmas suddenly seemed much more traditional than we were expecting. In fact, while we were enjoying Christmas dinner, a rare Arizona phenomenon occurred. It began to snow! According to newspaper accounts, this was the first snow in Phoenix on Christmas in 50 years.

So, instead of swimming, David and Amy spent the rest of Christmas day with their cousins fashioning the light white powder into a dirty snowman.

Before we started our trip, Jack reluctantly agreed that we wouldn't burden our parents with the results of the latest scan. Consequently, we found many other topics of conversation with my family, and, for the first time in months, I was able to divert my mind away from my illness. As a result, our trip took on a beneficial effect for me beyond just the social and family aspects. In many ways it was as therapeutic for my psyche as the chemicals hopefully were for my body. It was, one might say, just what the doctor ordered. However, the recurring pain in my right rib cage when I moved a certain way was a constant reminder of what lay ahead.

A couple of days after Christmas, we started the second leg of our journey to San Antonio. I have always loved Texas ever since my first visit there in 1959. It was a place where I could be reasonably warm all winter without the congestion of thousands of winter visitors or "snow birds." And Jack's large, wonderful family always made me feel at home.

On our first weekend in Texas, Jack's family held a reunion attended by his parents, sisters, nieces, nephews, and any other immediate family member in a 200-mile radius. David and Amy were somewhat overwhelmed by the numbers but happy to get to know more about their Dad's relatives.

Since Jack had broached the subject of retirement from the Navy before we left Maryland, I suggested that we look at San Antonio real estate while we were there. After all, San Antonio boasted of having two of the finest military hospitals in the country—Brooke Army Medical Center and Wilford Hall USAF Medical Center. All three of his sisters lived there as well. And, if anything happened to me, I knew they would treat David and Amy like their own children and provide Jack with the emotional support he would need.

After searching for a couple of days, we finally found a lovely English Tudor style home in a new community which suited our taste and pocketbook. Situated on a half-acre, oak-tree studded lot, the custom-built house featured an antique brick exterior and a cedar shake roof. Although it was essentially complete, the builder had left certain parts to be customized to the purchaser's specifications.

As much as we liked this house, we were in no position to sign an earnest money contract while we were in Texas. We still had a home in Rockville, and Jack had not yet requested retirement from the Navy.

David and Amy were overjoyed at the prospect of moving to Texas. They were completely fascinated with the wildlife of the state—from the cotton-tail rabbits in the back yard of what they hoped would be our new home to the white-tailed deer which grazed across the street at dusk. They were even charmed by the smaller fauna, and they amused themselves by temporarily

The Fat Lady Hasn't Sung

enslaving the green lizards (which inhabited the shrubbery around buildings) by putting string leashes around their necks.

Inevitably, the time came for our vacation to end, and I had to face the reality of resuming our efforts of trying to slow down the rapid growth of my tumors.

The day after we returned home, I checked in with Dr. Lokey. He was quite anxious to start the new chemotherapy cycle after my longer-than-normal respite. As soon as the results of my finger stick came back from the lab showing my white blood count had returned to acceptable levels, Dr. Lokey prepared to start my injection. He explained that in order to be able to deliver what he considered adequate doses of Adriamycin, he was going to inject a larger-than-ever dose of that drug now, followed only by Vincristine the next day. Then, for the next seven days, I would have to take Procarbazine pills by mouth.

Aside from using a larger syringe, Dr. Lokey's preparations for my first shot followed the usual pattern. Within seconds of the Adriamycin entering my veins, however, this time I experienced a different taste in my mouth as bitter as gall.

Dr. Lokey must have noticed the sour expression on my face. "What's wrong, Mary? You look like you just bit into a lemon."

"Try dandelion! It tastes just like dandelion juice!"

"How would you know what that tasted like?" Dr. Lokey asked with a puzzled expression.

"I haven't been out grazing recently. But I ate one when I was a kid. And that's a taste you never forget."

"Maybe they added some dandelion wine to this Adriamycin batch," he quipped, trying to humor me.

During our Christmas vacation, I almost managed to eradicate the horrible memories of my violent nausea and vomiting. But, true to form, within an hour of my injection, the terrible retching returned with a vengeance.

As soon as Jack returned to work after our trip he looked into the Navy's retirement procedures. When he found out he could retire at the end of June, he put in his papers to start the administrative wheels rolling.

Simultaneously, we listed our home with the same real-estate agent who helped us find it four years earlier. We obviously priced it too low because it sold to the first couple who saw it the day after the listing was filed. Surprisingly, they didn't need it right away, and we agreed on a June settlement.

This rapid-fire chain of events freed us up to try to work out a deal on that San Antonio house we had liked so much. Jack negotiated by telephone and finally managed to bring the builder down to about the same price as we were getting for our Rockville home. But in the trade, we were getting a house with many more amenities, more room, and much more quality throughout.

It appeared that my long desire to live in Texas was going to be realized at last!

As soon as my current chemotherapy cycle was over, I returned by prearrangement to Dr. Beatty at the radiation therapy clinic to begin treatment to my rib. His enthusiasm for his medical specialty had not waned since our last meeting. He explained that he was planning to use cobalt again and that the treatments would run for about ten days. After examining me physically, I fully expected Dr. Beatty to produce his red indelible marker to make the benchmarks on my body for the radiation bombardment to follow.

Instead, he surprised me. "We're going to tattoo you, Mary, so we can see where to direct the rays."

I thought Dr. Beatty was kidding me, so I decided to play along. "Instead of the usual 'Mom' tattoo, could you make mine read 'Dad?'"

"Seriously, we need very precise marks on that part of your body, Mary. We don't want to radiate and perhaps harm your internal organs."

I was beginning to realize Dr. Beatty was dead serious. "But do I really have to be tattooed?"

"We're just going to tattoo four dots which represent the corners of a rectangle. Besides, they'll probably fade over time."

In addition to his prowess with his red marker, I soon discovered Dr. Beatty's skill with a tattoo needle. After determining the rectangle to be radiated, he pricked in a dot of blue coloring matter at each corner.

When he finished making his marks, I looked down at my rib and saw the blue dots which were now permanently imbedded under my skin.

I thought whimsically to myself that after sixteen years of marriage to a Naval officer, with my tattoo I could now qualify as a member of the seafarers' society on my own.

Chapter Twenty-One

"Beware the ides of March," the Soothsayer warned Julius Caesar in Shakespeare's play.

Julius Caesar didn't heed the warning, but I should have.

The month of February and the first part of March were busy times for us.

After ten days of radiation to my right rib, Dr. Beatty decided I had absorbed enough rads to kill the tumor. Sure enough, the pain diminished after about three sessions and finally vanished after my eighth treatment. Once again, the cobalt spared me the severe skin burns of conventional radiation therapy. But my tattoo target was still completely intact and probably set permanently after the gamma-ray bombardment.

Shortly after my cobalt treatments were over, it was time again for the next chemotherapy cycle. Dr. Lokey kidded me before the Adriamycin injection that he had "spiked" my dose with dandelion wine. When he emptied the syringe into my vein, once more that distinctive bitter taste reminiscent of dandelions came to my mouth. The only possible explanation Dr. Lokey could offer for my new taste sensations was that my body chemistry had changed since my first injection of Adriamycin. But even though the taste was different, unfortunately, the all-too-familiar nausea and uncontrollable vomiting remained constant.

Between radiation and chemotherapy treatments, Jack and I also were busy making arrangements for settlement on our new home in Texas and planning our move in June. In addition, Jack applied for an instructor's position at San Antonio College. (Although his baccalaureate degree was in journalism, he later obtained a master's degree in management when our children were still infants by going to classes at night after work and on weekends.)

In preparation for my next chemotherapy cycle, Dr. Lokey scheduled me for a routine white blood count check and physical exam on March 15th—the "ides of March."

Everyone in the metropolitan Washington area must have had an appointment at Bethesda that day, I thought, as I inched along under overcast skies through row after row of parked cars in the patients' parking area. There was not a vacant spot to be had. With the time for my appointment at hand, in desperation I decided to park in the "north 40"—an overflow parking area some distance from the hospital, used primarily by employees and staff.

Despite the parking problem, I somehow made it to my appointment on time. Dr. Lokey saw me immediately and pronounced me ready for my next chemotherapy. In less than an hour, I was on my way again.

As I trudged past the hundreds of parked cars enroute to my distant spot at the far end of the lot, I was elated over the prospect of having some unexpected additional shopping time.

When I finally neared my car, the next thing I knew I was careening headlong toward the ground. My legs were unable to keep up with the momentum of my upper body, and I came crashing down on the macadam with the full impact on my left side.

As I rolled over onto my back and stared up at the gray sky, I thought, "Here we go again! How could this have happened?"

When I finally struggled to sit up, I knew without a doubt from the distinctive pain that I had broken my hip again.

The parking lot at that hour was as devoid of humans as the moon. But I knew I needed help, so I began to yell and whistle. After waiting futilely for about ten minutes for some sign of life to appear, I realized I had two choices. I could wait another hour for the hospital shift change, or I could attempt to make it to the car on my own.

I decided to opt for the latter. Inch by inch I dragged my body toward the car, as sharp pains radiated down my leg with each movement. When I finally got within reach of the door, I used the handle like a trapeze for pulling my body upward. This enabled me to unlock the door and swing it open. With access to the steering wheel, I repeated my circus act by pulling myself onto the seat. By now, the pain was almost overwhelming.

Somehow, I started my car and drove to the emergency room entrance. (Thank goodness for automatic transmissions!) I honked my horn for several minutes before a corpsman with a look of exasperation on his youthful face appeared at the door.

"You can't park here, lady! This is the ambulance entrance," he yelled curtly.

"I'm sorry, but I've broken my hip," I replied emotionally. The pain now was almost intolerable.

My response at least got his attention, and he came over to my side of the car. "So you've broken your hip, have you?" he asked as he looked me over at close range. "I'm so sure," he mumbled under his breath, saying something to the effect that young women don't break hips.

I must have convinced him of the severity of my injury, however, since he disappeared abruptly and reappeared within seconds, pushing an empty wheelchair.

By now the discomfort was constant, and I can't recall a more painful transfer to a wheelchair. Once inside, the corpsman borrowed my keys and moved my car to a legitimate parking space.

While I waited for the emergency room staff to see me, other than my gnawing pain, my main concern was to call Jack to let him know I wouldn't be able to meet David and Amy when they got home from school.

X-rays confirmed my provisional diagnosis. My left hip was fractured again.

As soon as the emergency room doctors determined the nature of my injury, they quickly dispatched me to the orthopedic ward for admission.

When Mrs. Collins, the orthopedic head nurse, saw me, her eyes lit up and she ran over to greet me.

"Mary Walker! Am I glad to see you! What are you doing here?"

When I told her about my encounter with the parking lot pavement, she offered words of comfort. But she quickly resumed expressing her delight about my being there.

"I have the perfect room for you, Mary. Your new roommate is terribly depressed. But I know you're just the person to cheer her up."

"You've got to be kidding," I began. "I need someone to cheer *me* up about now."

"Mary, you're ideal for this job. You're the most upbeat person I know. Please do it for me."

I reluctantly agreed, not that I had many options since Mrs. Collins made the room assignments anyhow.

Mrs. Collins pushed me to my new room and introduced me to Lisa Kerr. Lisa was a pretty girl in her late twenties with a yuppie countenance about her even before the word had been coined. She looked like she would be much more at home in tennis attire at a country club than in pajamas in a military hospital bed. Her right leg had been crushed in several places in an automobile accident, and the corrective surgery to repair her bones had been slow to heal.

Lisa acknowledged my introduction with a faint smile and turned over on her side, facing the windows, in the opposite direction of my bed.

I wasn't too upset by Lisa's aloofness since my main concern was to get some relief for my broken hip. Within minutes after transferring to my bed, a pair of orthopedic technicians arrived to place my left leg in traction and to install a set of monkey bars. Mrs. Collins gave me a shot of pain medication, and within a few minutes I was resting rather comfortably.

I looked over toward Lisa's end of the room, and it was obvious from the accumulation of greeting cards and personal objects that she had been hospitalized for a long time.

A poster-sized portrait of a basset hound covered the wall at the foot of her bed. The name "Penelope" was printed across the top of the photograph. Penelope's characteristic sad eyes and long ears reminded me of another basset hound at another place and time.

When Jack was stationed in Puerto Rico, we were invited to a New Year's eve party at the home of the commanding officer and his wife, Captain and Mrs. Goren.

The party was quite formal, and the Goren's spacious quarters were bedecked with the traditional decorations for the occasion. Mrs. Goren, a short and obese person who weighed at least 200 pounds, had a fondness for low, Japanese-style tables. Several of these tables were strategically located around her living room, each laden with trays of hors d'oeuvres and bowls of nuts.

As the 30-odd guests talked and visited, the Goren's tri-colored basset hound, Clem, surreptitiously slithered around and under the tables. No one seemed to notice Clem's party-crashing antics except Jack and me. Clem seemed especially fond of the table next to the guest of honor, a visiting admiral from Washington, D.C. As the admiral talked to a couple of senior officers' wives, he methodically reached down occasionally without looking to a wooden monkey-pod bowl filled with salted peanuts and grabbed a handful of nuts. After each reach by the admiral, Clem came out from under the table, extended his long, pink, salivating tongue into the peanut bowl, and gulped down a mouthful. After the admiral and Clem alternated back and forth several times, the bowl was soon emptied without the admiral ever realizing with whom he had shared his snack.

Flush with his success at the peanut bowl, Clem waddled over to another table. Sure enough, no one noticed Clem gulp down a couple of finger sandwiches as animated conversationalists vied for the same food with the stealthy canine.

Finally, Clem got a little too bold when he placed his two front paws on the dining room table in order to reach a tasty morsel. Mrs. Goren spied her brazen basset from across the room just as he began licking the rolled anchovies.

"Clem! Get down from that table!" Mrs. Goren screamed as she lunged her corpulent body toward her erring dog.

Clem got the message loud and clear. In his haste to comply with his master's order, he snagged the dewclaw on his forepaw in a hole in the lace tablecloth and pulled the cloth and all the table's contents onto the floor. Mrs. Goren couldn't stop her forward momentum in time to prevent her from stepping squarely on the pile of food and dishes. Whatever survived the fall, she smashed to smithereens like a bull in a china shop.

Clem made a hasty exit toward the kitchen, with Mrs. Goren yelling and screaming as she thundered along after him.

Jack and I could hardly contain ourselves at the wonderful comedy of the occasion where one innocent-looking basset hound had totally disrupted such a grand social gathering. Judging from Mrs. Goren's demeanor, we were pretty sure that by the time the clock struck midnight, Clem was in the dog house, literally *and* physically.

I don't know if the old adage that no germs can live in a dog's mouth is true or not. But on that New Year's eve, I'm sure there were a lot of people who hoped it was.

My contemplation of the past ended as Jack hurried in and embraced me, fresh from having met David and Amy after school and taking them to Hilda Ponder's. Naturally, he was upset about my fall and curious to learn the details.

I had scarcely finished telling Jack about the events of the afternoon when two unfamiliar doctors appeared.

Introducing themselves as Doctors Blake and Jones, orthopedic residents, they explained that Dr. Slimmons and the rest of the orthopedic surgical staff were in San Francisco for a week-long medical convention. The only orthopedic doctors left at Bethesda were residents and interns.

Both doctors strongly recommended surgery to repair my fractured hip. They also cautioned against waiting until the regular staff returned in six days.

Jack and I were in a quandary about what to do. On the one hand, we wanted Dr. Slimmons to be available to supervise any surgery. But on the other, we were uneasy about waiting so long to have the hip fixed.

After a long deliberation, I finally decided to have the surgery as soon as the two residents could make the arrangements, which turned out to be the next day. They explained that they intended to "offset the femur and secure it with Jewett nails," which was standard procedure in such cases.

Before Jack left for the evening, I asked him to call oncology and talk to Dr. Lokey about postponing the next chemotherapy treatment.

During Jack's visit and while the doctors were present, my roommate, Lisa, busied herself fixing her nails and otherwise appearing to be uninterested in my case.

As soon as Jack was gone, she turned toward me. "Mary, I heard you mention oncology. Who has cancer?"

"I do," I replied unemotionally. "And while I'm here in the hospital, I'll probably have to have a round of chemotherapy. I hope that won't bother you too much."

My revelation seemed to cause her veil of aloofness to lift almost immediately, and she began warming up to me. After a month of feeling sorry for herself, she finally realized someone else might be worse off than she was.

She asked me about other aspects of my illness and seemed fascinated by my progression from bed to wheelchair to crutches to cane to walking again without any support. I assured her (trying to reassure myself) that my current problem was a slight detour on the road to complete recovery.

Early the next morning I boarded the gurney, which wheeled me to the OR again. As the automatic doors swung open and the bright lights and chilled air hit me, second thoughts about my decision began to engulf me. I wondered if I should have waited for Dr. Slimmons and the first string instead of going with the substitutes.

Chapter Twenty-Two

"That's what I call perfect placement," Dr. Blake beamed as he busied himself at the X-ray viewer in my room.

I was still groggy from the surgery, having just been released from the recovery room. But I was alert enough to see the images Dr. Blake was raving about.

"Just look at those nails! Dr. Jewett couldn't have done it better himself."

The X-rays revealed two square-headed nails, about four inches long, extending through the top of my femur into the neck and head of the bone.

Even though my eyes weren't focusing clearly, I knew immediately I didn't share Dr. Blake's enthusiasm.

"Are you sure the nails weren't designed by Dr. Frankenstein instead of Dr. Jewett? They look like something from the Dark Ages," I countered as Dr. Blake continued to gaze at his handiwork.

"You're lucky they're on the inside, Mrs. Walker." Dr. Blake obviously was referring to the medieval-looking torture devices which orthopedic surgeons are notorious for using on the outside of the body.

Dr. Blake's X-rays were still on display when Jack returned. After he was sure I had come through the surgery successfully, he had gone back to work and then home to meet the children after school before coming back to the hospital.

Dr. Blake seemed eager to show his orthopedic masterpiece to Jack. But from Jack's facial expressions, I got the unmistakable message that he wasn't too impressed either.

Jack stayed on for another hour or so, filling me in on activities at home and getting updated on my condition.

Jack couldn't have been gone fifteen minutes when a male voice resounded from the doorway. "Have I got a treat for you! It's pizza time!"

The voice belonged to Dr. Bob Kerr, Lisa's husband. Dr. Kerr was a tall, thin, handsome man in his early thirties, who wore a Clark Gable-style mustache. He was assigned as a staff dentist at Bethesda, and I had met him briefly the night before. Since he was on staff, he was exempt from normal visiting hours.

He strode briskly into the room carrying two containers of pizza and wearing a huge smile. From what I could determine, his routine was to surprise Lisa with a different treat each night in what up to this point had been a futile effort to cheer her up.

When Dr. Kerr offered me a couple of large pieces, I declined on the basis of my queasy stomach. But I told him I'd take a rain check.

For the next two hours, Bob Kerr entertained Lisa and me with his non-stop anecdotes about life on the staff at Bethesda.

Each evening Dr. Kerr continued his repertory of surprises. One night it was homemade ice cream sundaes, complete with all the toppings. On another, fresh popped popcorn—my favorite snack—was the treat of the evening. Of course, he always included me in both the conversation and the food. Between Dr. Kerr's surprise parties and my daily conversations with Lisa, her despondency began yielding to mild optimism.

Three days after my surgery, I made my first trip to physical therapy to begin to work my way back to using crutches. Two therapists assisted me as I stood up on my right leg and positioned the crutches under my arms. As I moved forward and placed weight on my offset left hip, I experienced the strangest sensation with my right leg—my "good" one—I had ever felt. When I tried to move my right leg through to complete the stepping motion, it seemed too long—far too long—to finish the step. It felt like anything but a leg as I dragged it along the floor.

"My leg feels like an elephant's trunk!" I exclaimed as I struggled with my newest dilemma. "My right leg must be three inches longer than it was before my surgery!"

The therapists laughed and assured me my right leg hadn't grown any in four days.

Three days later, Dr. Slimmons re-appeared during morning rounds, carrying a packet of X-rays.

"Welcome back, Dr. Slimmons!" I greeted him happily. "How was your trip to San Francisco? Did you leave your heart there?"

"Hello, Mary! My trip was fine. I only left my money. I understand you had a problem while I was gone."

"Yeah, I did what you warned me not to do—I fell. But my biggest problem right now is my right leg. It seems so much longer than the left one. Every time I go to physical therapy, I'm like Dumbo—at least my right leg feels like his trunk."

Dr. Slimmons told his colleagues to continue their rounds without him as he re-lit his pipe. He then pulled several X-rays from the envelope and positioned them on the viewer. I recognized them immediately upon seeing the square-headed nails. He drew deeply on his pipe as he studied the negatives and then smiled faintly as he responded. "Mary, your right leg hasn't changed. But your left leg is now about three inches shorter than it was. They had to 'offset,' or shorten, your femur bone approximately three inches to provide stability for the nails."

"But how am I ever going to manage? My right leg drags the ground when I try to walk with crutches."

"We need to put a lift on your left shoe. Have Jack buy you a pair of sturdy, 'sensible' shoes, and we'll measure you and install the lift here at our brace shop."

Dr. Slimmons could tell from my expression that I wasn't enthralled over the prospect of wearing old-fashioned, built-up orthopedic shoes the rest of my life.

"I'm sorry, Mary. I wish I had been here when the decision was made." Dr. Slimmons fidgeted with the X-rays as he searched for his words. "The procedure my residents did was done right—they just didn't do the *right* procedure. They should have gone ahead and replaced your hip."

The next day Jack showed up carrying a shopping bag. He smiled impishly as he pulled out a shoe box. "You're really going to like these shoes, Mary. They're the latest fashion at the Red Cross Shoe store."

Jack removed a pair of navy blue, lace-up shoes with heavy soles and thick heels. They reminded me of some matronly fashion of a bygone era.

"Oh, no!" I reacted. "I'm going to look just like Rosa Klebb in those clodhoppers. All I need are knife blades extending from my toes!"

Jack looked puzzled. Unlike me, he was not a big Ian Fleming fan, so he was not familiar with most of James Bond's nemeses. But Lisa, having seen the shoes and overheard our conversation, erupted with laughter.

"Oh, Jack, you know who that is!" Lisa joined in, hardly able to contain her amusement. Rosa Klebb was the SMERSH agent who attacked James Bond with her spiked shoes in *From Russia, With Love.*"

Within a couple of days my built-up shoe was ready, complete with its three inches of additional sole and heel. My first impression, other than looking like Carmen Miranda in one of her costumes, was that it resembled a lead weight. Indeed, all that additional leather must have weighed several pounds. But during my next PT session, my right leg had lost its seeming elephantine characteristics, and I began to make true progress ambulating with crutches.

My real aversion to the kind of shoes I was now forced to wear probably went back to an April night in 1963 in Rome.

Jack and I had obtained tickets to the Teatro dell'Opera's performance of Verdi's *Il Trovatore*, featuring the American baritone Cornell MacNeil and an all Italian cast, none of whom were internationally known. We had excellent aisle seats in the center orchestra. Unfortunately, the occupant of the seat next to me arrived to claim her spot just as Maestro Tullio Serafin gave the downbeat for the ominous drum rolls opening the first scene. After making a big disturbance finding the right row, she presented, as is customary in Europe, her bloated abdomen, cinched in by her gold lamé dress, to Jack's face. (Members of an audience when moving between rows of seats, always face toward the seated person, never extending their backsides to those seated as Americans usually do.)

Since there was no way the latecomer could fit between Jack and the seat in front of him, he rose and quickly exited to the aisle. I wasn't so fortunate. By the time I could stand up, our plump companion was already moving ponderously down the row toward the empty seat. Even though I pushed back on my upright seat as hard as I could, her belly made full contact with my body, and momentarily she seemed to be stuck. Simultaneous with our body contact, she stepped on both my feet, almost as if by design, and it seemed I got the full brunt of her gargantuan weight. At that moment I got my first whiff of her "fragrance." It was a curious mixture of aromas including a strong, cheap perfume, body odor, garlic, halitosis, moth balls, and mildew. Mercifully, in a twisting movement, she finally freed herself and moved on to her seat. As she plopped down, she gave a huge sigh, and the entire row shook.

As soon as I regained the feeling in my feet, I caught a glimpse of the shoes which had been the source of my torment. Sure enough! They were a pair of "sensible," lace-up, old-fashioned orthopedic shoes—about size ten!

My seat neighbor was wearing a stole decorated with what seemed like at least a dozen fox heads along its ample girth. One head seemed to be resting on my shoulder, its beady, agate eyes staring at me throughout the opera. In the second act when the

Anvil Chorus began, my seat mate started to keep time with the swinging hammers of the stage Gypsies. With each clank against the metal forges onstage, she responded by thumping her silver-headed cane against the ancient wooden opera house floor.

Later in Act II when MacNeil completed his beautiful aria, *Il balen del suo sorriso*, modest applause emerged from the audience along with a few *"bravos,"* mostly from Jack. The woman in the orthopedic shoes hissed her disapproval through purple painted lips. Each time one of the Italian members of the cast completed an aria or ensemble, the audience erupted with loud applause and numerous shouts of approval. It was clear to us that, unlike La Scala, the Rome Opera was showing its provincialism by "rooting for the home team" and providing ample evidence of the continued existence of a claque system.

Just before the end of the final scene my tormentor in the next seat began rocking back and forth. When she built up enough momentum, she raised her body and stood. Before I could respond to her final lunge, she began pushing toward the aisle, trying to get a head start on the crowd. Once more she positioned her orthopedic shoes squarely on top of my feet in a repeat of the fiasco at the opera's opening. By the time the final curtain fell, she was halfway up the aisle. During curtain calls, I was applauding more out of a sense of relief than approbation of the singers. Thank God, I thought, I won't have to endure those shoes again.

My physical therapy sessions continued to go well, and my progress seemed to inspire Lisa to try harder. We even scheduled our PT visits at the same time to provide encouragement for each other.

A few days later I received word to report to the oncology clinic. I knew that my chemotherapy treatment was overdue, so it was no surprise when Dr. Lokey suggested we resume treatment immediately.

"I wanted to get you started before you left the hospital," Dr. Lokey said as he readied the cranberry-colored syringe. "I've also ordered a bone scan to see if the increased doses are paying off."

Dr. Lokey seemed to have an exceptionally difficult time

finding a vein, and when he finally injected the medicine in the outside of the forearm, I felt an unusual stinging sensation.

The predictable vomiting started shortly after I returned to the room. After seeing me retch, it was obvious Lisa wasn't prepared to be around someone with the aftereffects of chemotherapy.

"Oh, Mary, I had no idea it was going to be this bad. What can I do to help?"

"It would be nice if you could ring the nurse when my basin needs emptying. It just takes time to run its course," I reassured her.

When the vomiting finally subsided, I became more aware of the burning sensation in my arm.

After a restless night I discovered that my forearm was inflamed and swollen. As soon as I showed my arm to Mrs. Collins, she summoned Dr. Lokey.

When Dr. Lokey arrived, he knew immediately what had happened. "Oh, no! The needle must have nicked the other side of your vein. The drug has infiltrated the surrounding tissue."

"Does that make the treatment ineffective?"

"No, your body will absorb it. But we must act aggressively to prevent the drug from coming through your arm and making an open sore. Those types of sores are very difficult if not impossible to heal."

Dr. Lokey ordered around-the-clock hot packs to be applied on the area along with cortisone cream.

The burning sensation had almost disappeared by the time I reported for my bone scan. While I was confident about the results, Jack remained very apprehensive.

When I returned to my room, Lisa and Bob were packing to leave.

"Mary, I got the green light to go home. I wish you were leaving too," Lisa began, revealing her mixed emotions.

"Don't worry. I won't be far behind you," I reassured her as I swung onto the bed.

When Lisa had finished packing she crutched over to my bed to say goodbye.

"It's been wonderful having you as a roommate, Mary. I was so depressed before you came, but you were an inspiration for me and made my stay almost fun."

"I didn't do anything, Lisa. You did it all yourself. We'll keep in touch at physical therapy as outpatients. Be careful, and give Penelope a hug for me."

The next day Dr. Lokey informed me that the bone scan showed no new lesions. The higher chemotherapy dosages apparently were working.

When my chemotherapy cycle ended, I was released with instructions to continue the hot packs and cream.

Once again, I felt I was bouncing back from adversity.

Chapter Twenty-Three

"How much for the ski stuff, Mrs. Walker?"

The voice came from Jimmy Patton, one of the neighborhood kids.

"I don't know. Make me an offer I can't refuse. I'll throw in the skis, boots, poles, and a pair of ice skates for good measure."

One thing I knew for certain was that I wasn't going to need winter sports gear in Texas with my offset femur and me on crutches. During my high school and college years in Minnesota, I had numerous occasions to use my equipment. But since our marriage, I had used my ice skates only once on a frozen pond in Bremerhaven. Although I wasn't a Sonja Henie, I think I impressed Jack that I could stay on my feet.

Jimmy reached into his pocket and pulled out several crumpled dollar bills. Without counting the money, I accepted Jimmy's offer.

Our garage sale was a huge success in getting rid of items Jack and I didn't want to move to Texas. Financially, however, we were lucky to realize almost enough to pay for a dinner for the four of us.

The Fat Lady Hasn't Sung

Time went quickly after I returned home from the hospital. Maneuvering around on crutches and dragging my built-up shoe slowed me down some in our race to get everything done before our move to Texas in June.

A couple of weeks after I returned home, Jack was summoned to Texas for interviews at the college where he had applied to teach. He reluctantly agreed to leave me for a few days since he was so anxious to secure that job. When the kids and I met him at the airport upon his return, I could tell from his big grin that things had gone well. Sure enough, a week later the department chairman called to inform Jack that he had been selected for the full-time, tenure track position of instructor in management, effective the first of August.

While he was in San Antonio, Jack also signed the final settlement papers on our new home.

Things were starting to fall into place. Barring some new medical setback, my life-long dream of living in Texas seemed to be within our grasp.

During my next chemotherapy treatment, Dr. Lokey examined my drug burn and decided I could finally stop the hot packs and special cream. He confirmed what I already had decided. That ugly scar on my forearm—as angry and red as if I had been branded by a fiery hot poker—was going to be with me for the rest of my days.

Our last month in Washington was one of the most hectic of our lives. Our closest friends wined and dined us to wish us Godspeed on our embarking into an uncertain future—no one knowing if I would live to see them ever again. The gang at Jack's office threw a series of retirement parties for him, presenting him with plaques and mementoes of his 20-year career in the Navy. His most treasured gift from his peers was an official lone-star flag of the State of Texas.

During this busy time, our dog, Snoopy, began throwing up at frequent intervals. At first, we noticed it about once a week; but finally, it became an almost daily occurrence. The veterinarian readily diagnosed the problem as infected anal glands and recommended immediate surgery. Since three days of traveling with a vomiting dog in the back seat was unacceptable, we decided to go ahead with the eleventh-hour surgery. Snoopy breezed through the operation uneventfully, although the vet cautioned that drainage from the area could continue for a while.

When the time arrived for the movers to pack out our household effects, as luck would have it, Dr. Lokey also had scheduled me for my last chemotherapy treatment at Bethesda.

When I reported to his clinic, Dr. Lokey was all prepared. My drugs were drawn and in readiness for my injections. In addition, Dr. Lokey gave me a copy of a letter he had sent to the chief of Oncology Service of Brooke Army Medical Center (BAMC) in San Antonio. When he finished administering the chemotherapy, Dr. Lokey bade me an emotional farewell and asked me to keep in touch. While waiting for the elevator en route to my car and wondering if I would see him again, I opened the envelope and glanced over his letter. It read in part:

> Mrs. Mary Walker is a 38-year-old Caucasian female with a diagnosis of histiocytic lymphoma of the bone. CDR Walker has recently retired, and the family will be moving to your area in mid-June. I understand that you have agreed to assume responsibility for Mrs. Walker's oncologic care. I hope that the following will serve as an outline of her rather complicated disease course. . .

Dr. Lokey presented a lengthy recapitulation of my medical history since May of 1973, including all the major surgical procedures, diagnostic tests, and various treatments.

He concluded the letter with this observation:

> . . .I foresee several potential problems in the future management of this patient. Marrow reserves are significantly limited by previous radio and chemotherapy. Dosage modifications or even a period of delay without therapy may be needed in the future. The patient's peripheral veins are in poor condition, and have been significantly depleted by previous

chemotherapy efforts. There is significant structural instability of both femurs with the probable necessity for further orthopedic intervention...

Both Mrs. Walker and her husband are extremely pleasant, cooperative people to deal with. She is well motivated, and despite a multitude of complications has maintained an active family and social life. I feel certain that you will enjoy your association with her. If I can be of help in her management please contact me...

    Sincerely,
    Julian L. Lokey
    LCDR, MC USNR
    Staff, Hematology/Oncology Branch

I arrived home as usual just before the nausea hit. But this time our house was swarming with movers. One man was working in the family room, another in the basement, and Jack was in the dining room supervising a third packer as he methodically wrapped paper around each piece of crystal and packed it into a large cardboard box.

By the time I crutched upstairs and got into bed, the first wave of vomiting hit with its usual intensity. Jack was there to comfort me and empty my pink pan each time I got sick, dividing his time the rest of the day between me and the movers.

When I was finally ready for my root-beer chaser, our home had been totally transformed. Sealed cardboard boxes, often stacked several deep, were scattered throughout each room.

Paintings and wall hangings which had adorned our walls were now carefully resting in wooden crates. Larger pieces of furniture were tagged and inventoried, ready to be loaded into the moving van the next day along with all the boxes and crates. Our home was now a mere house.

With everything packed except our suitcases and clothes for our trip to Texas, it was time now for us to vacate as well. Having anticipated our moving difficulties, the Ponders invited us to spend our last couple of days in the Washington area with them.

With me on one arm, and carrying my well-used pink pan in the other, Jack led me the hundred some odd feet to the Ponder's home. Hilda turned over one of her two lovely master bedroom suites to Jack and me and guest rooms for David and Amy.

While I recuperated from the rest of my chemotherapy at the Ponders, Jack spent every spare moment cleaning our house and making it ready for the walk-through inspection by the purchasers and their real-estate agent.

Finally, early on a bright June morning, we were ready to leave on our long-awaited trip to Texas.

Snoopy was perched in her basket in the back seat, her tongue drooped in a happy grin, flanked on each side by David and Amy.

Since Snoopy was still draining from her recent surgery, Jack improvised a way to keep her basket reasonably clean. Using his old Jockey briefs, he slipped them on upside down over her hindquarters, pushing her upright tail through the fly opening in front. We were driving our family automobile—a 1972 Chevrolet Impala—and towing Jack's Vega commuter car. We must have looked like modern-day Okies in our two-car caravan, with me on crutches, two kids bouncing on the back seat, and a dog wearing men's underwear.

The first part of our journey went smoothly except for a nervous Snoopy whose panting and salivating on the kids kept them on edge. After a couple of hundred miles, Snoopy finally got used to the riding motion and went to sleep. As it turned out, Snoopy's position between David and Amy was a fortuitous event, providing a buffer during the next three days between two tired and restless youngsters.

We decided to stop for the night when we reached Bristol, Virginia, since going on to Knoxville, Tennessee would have been too difficult. After sitting in one position for several hours, my hips were starting to stiffen and cause me more discomfort than usual.

Jack called his sister, Nora, in San Antonio to let her know we were on our way. During the conversation, his face grew longer and longer as she told him about the latest crisis. It seems they had turned on the air conditioning in our home in Texas in anticipation of our arrival. As is the custom in many newer homes in Texas, the heating/air conditioning units were installed in the attic. The workmen, however, had failed to connect the condensation drain pipe to the sewer, and all the water was collecting in the ceiling. When the weight of the accumulated water became excessive, the ceiling of David's bedroom came crashing down, soaking the carpet and scattering insulation and debris about the room. Nora already had notified the builder, and work had begun to remedy the situation. Surprisingly, Jack was rather calm in telling us about our latest misfortune. After so much life and death involvement, material damage which could be repaired seemed rather insignificant by comparison.

Our second day of travel was uneventful, except I had to spend more time entertaining the children. Their initial enthusiasm for the trip had long since waned, and their boredom resulted in constant arguments and spats. Although Jack stopped often for rest and meals, I was experiencing more and more hip pain. By the time we arrived in Vicksburg, Mississippi, we were all ready for a break from the car and a good night's sleep.

When we got to the Texas-Louisiana border on the third day of travel, Jack posed all of us, including Snoopy, next to the stone monument in the shape of Texas (which is always present at every highway point of entry in the state) and took pictures. By now my hips were bothering me so much that it was hard to smile for the photographs.

We arrived in San Antonio later that day and went directly to Nora's house where we had a wonderful dinner and spent the first night. By applying pressure on the builder, she somehow had managed to get all the ceiling repairs completed by the time we arrived.

Early the next morning, by prearrangement, the moving van which left Rockville four days earlier pulled up in front of our new home, and workmen began unloading furniture and cartons of household effects. Although the movers were more than willing to help us unpack, about all we could do during the off-loading process was to direct items to the right room, since we weren't sure where everything was going ourselves.

Two hours later, the van was empty. But our home was piled high with dozens of cartons, crates, and larger items of furniture. The task of unpacking that mass and arranging everything in its proper place seemed insurmountable. Jack's first objective was to get all our beds set up so we could sleep that night. I tried my best to help, but my hip pain was now so intense that I could only stay on my feet a few minutes at a time.

As Jack finished tightening the bolts on our bed rails, he emerged from his prone position on the carpet covered with sweat. He strode over to where I was seated on a camphor-wood linen chest at the foot of the bed and bent over to kiss me. "Well, Mary darlin', here we are at last—in Texas in our own home!"

The constant pain in my hips and the frustration I felt at not being able to help more finally overwhelmed me as tears welled up in my eyes. "Oh, Jack," I sobbed, "I'm in such awful shape. My legs are killing me. I'm never going to be able to enjoy this beautiful house!"

CHAPTER TWENTY-FOUR

Armed with Dr. Lokey's letter, a thick file of X-rays, and my medical record, I reported to the oncology clinic at BAMC.

Even though it had been 15 years since I got my last-minute inoculations there prior to going to Puerto Rico, the old Army medical center hadn't changed much. The main hospital was housed in a venerable seven-story, brick building. But more than half of the various clinics and wards, including oncology and orthopedics, were located in Beach Pavilion, a rambling, multi-winged building of Spanish architecture which reportedly had served as a barracks and stable for cavalry soldiers of a bygone era.

I scarcely had time to recover from the long crutching journey from the parking lot when my name was called. The source of the sound was an athletically-built black man in his mid-thirties. His handsome, clean-shaven face was accented by a quick, sincere smile. By his demeanor alone, I would have known that he was an oncologist. Dr. Deas introduced himself and led me into his cramped but orderly office. He explained that they had received Dr. Lokey's letter, and he had been assigned as my new oncologist. Dr. Deas reviewed my recent medical history and gave me a quick physical exam. He also took a finger stick to determine my white blood count and then headed for the lab.

After a few minutes Dr. Deas returned to his office with the blood test results. "Your count is still quite low from your last chemotherapy at Bethesda. We're going to have to watch it closely each week until we can start your treatments here."

I wasn't surprised by the low blood count, but I was concerned about my recent intense hip pain. "Do you think my pain is new cancer-related activity, Dr. Deas?"

"I don't think so, but let's find out," Dr. Deas said as he picked up the phone. In less than a minute, he completed his conversation, and, with an empathic smile, turned to me. "You have an appointment this afternoon with Dr. Jewell in orthopedics."

It now was becoming increasingly difficult to walk even short distances with my crutches. En route to the orthopedic clinic, I had to stop three times to help ease the progressive pain in both hips.

Precisely at the appointed time, Dr. Jewell introduced himself and escorted me to his neatly-appointed office. His desk was clear of paper and files, but an adjoining table displayed some of the paraphernalia of his medical specialty. After a short series of questions, he began peering at my old X-rays through wire-rimmed spectacles. His demeanor was very businesslike and formal, if not aloof. He reminded me of a scholarly professor of English I had at Mankato State. During a brief physical exam he seemed surprised at my limited range of motion in both hips. He ordered new X-rays and blood work and told me to report back Monday.

Between my visits to BAMC, Jack and I continued to unpack our household effects and get a bit more settled each day. My pain was constant, however, and any prolonged standing or walking had become almost unbearable. In spite of the pain, at my insistence, we invited Jack's parents as our first dinner guests after we were reasonably well settled. Jack started cooking the chicken on our indoor grill and asked me to turn it at mid-point while he picked up his mother and father. I'm glad no one was there to see me writhe in agony from just standing for those few minutes. My hip pain was every bit as intense now as it was earlier when the cancer was eating away at my bones.

I reported back to Dr. Jewell on Monday as instructed, but this time I had to wait a while until he returned from the operating room. He was still in his green operating garb when he strode briskly into his office.

"Hello, Mrs. Walker. Sorry to keep you waiting." His mien, while still formal, seemed to have mellowed a bit since our first meeting. "I've studied your new X-rays carefully, and I now know why you're in such pain."

"Oh, good. Is there anything that can be done for it?"

Dr. Jewell took my new X-rays out of their folder and began arranging them in sequential order on his viewer. He pointed to the first one.

"This is your left hip. The previous fracture shows nonunion. Also—and this must be causing unbearable pain—the Jewett nail is displaced into the acetabular rim."

While I wouldn't have been able to decipher his words, it was clear from the X-ray that the previous break had not healed. And one of the nails Dr. Blake had been so proud of had pierced into the hip joint, with its sharp point scraping inside the cup-shaped cavity of the pelvis each time I moved my leg.

I was so relieved that my pain was mechanically induced, rather than cancerously, that I could only sit in silence.

Dr. Jewell moved on to the next X-ray. "Now this is your right hip. Once again, there is non-union of the femoral neck fracture, and one of the nails they used to secure it has broken."

By now I was getting used to his vocabulary as I clearly saw the unhealed old fracture and the broken nail. But I was puzzled by what I was seeing. "How did my hips get so bad so quickly?"

Dr. Jewell continued to study the X-rays. "I would guess that the heightened activity involved in moving combined with three days of inactivity while riding to Texas caused both hips essentially to collapse."

"I can see I'm a mess. What do you recommend?"

"I don't think we can successfully patch you up anymore. I

recommend replacing both hips. But if we're going to do that, we need to move fast to prevent that Jewett nail from doing any more damage."

"I don't know much about hip replacements. Will that make me better?"

For the first time, Dr. Jewell gave a faint impression of a smile. "It won't make you any worse; but it could make you a whole lot better. I know for sure we can even up the length of your legs, and you can throw away that built up shoe."

He handed me some pamphlets about hip replacements. "Read this and talk it over with your husband. Then both of you come in Friday, and we'll discuss it. In the meantime, try not to move around any more than necessary."

Dr. Jewell's advice was hardly necessary as any standing or moving with my crutches had become almost unendurable.

When Jack and I returned Friday for our appointment with Dr. Jewell, we borrowed a wheelchair to help ease my journey through the hospital corridors.

I introduced Jack to Dr. Jewell who ushered us into his office in his usual business-like manner.

After a short silence, Dr. Jewell began the conversation. "Now that you've had a chance to think about total hip replacement, do you have any questions or thoughts about it?"

I flipped through the pamphlet he had given me earlier to the photograph of a woman riding a horse following her surgery. "From some of these accounts, hip replacement seems almost like a magic cure," I observed.

"Well, I can assure you it's not magic," Dr. Jewell countered. "But the technology has improved tremendously in the last ten years."

I glanced at the picture of the horse and rider once more. "I don't care about being able to ride horses or play tennis again. I just want to be free of pain and be able to walk. If I could lead a halfway normal life and be able to do things for and with my family again, I would be ecstatic."

A slight hint of a smile ventured across Dr. Jewell's face for only the second time since I had known him. "I believe we can achieve that, barring any complications." After a short pause, he continued. "So. Have you made a decision?"

I glanced at Jack who smiled with a look of reassurance. When I turned back to Dr. Jewell, I gave him my answer. "How soon can we schedule the surgery?"

"Before we do that, we need to discuss some things," Dr. Jewell said as he stood up and walked over to the table of prosthetic devices. He picked up a part which resembled something from an auto mechanics class and brought it over to where Jack and I were seated. "This is a Charnley-Mueller prosthesis, similar to the ones we'll be using for you."

Sensing the need for a little levity in this conversation, I couldn't resist observing: "And I'll bet this is named for Dr. Charnley and Dr. Mueller."

Dr. Jewell gave an acknowledging nod as he continued to explain the component. The device consisted of a stainless steel femoral "head," polished to a mirror-like finish, attached to a slightly curved and tapered steel shaft about six inches long. This rod was designed to fit down into the femur bone after the natural neck and head had been removed. The smooth head rotated in a plastic cup which Dr. Jewell explained would be glued into the pelvic cavity.

As Dr. Jewell continued to explain more of the details of my surgery, a strange feeling came over me. Shortly, those pieces of steel and plastic would become an integral part of my body. I knew I would never be the same again. The old adage about being held together by baling wire and straw sprung to mind. Realistically, of course, when I was struck by cancer, I knew my life had changed forever.

"Which hip are you doing first?" I finally asked. "I don't know which one is worse. They're both very painful."

"That's the other thing we need to talk about," Dr. Jewell responded. "Your oncologist is very reluctant to stop your chemotherapy treatments for two separate surgeries, fearing the disease could gain too much of a stronghold on you."

"But isn't that a chance we'll just have to take?" I asked, knowing that I would never be able to walk, even with crutches, in my present situation.

"Not if we do simultaneous bilateral total hip replacements."

Jack and I looked at each other with uncertainty. "Are you proposing to replace both hips at the *same* time?" Jack inquired incredulously.

"I'm suggesting that option—yes. Normally, we would *never* undertake such an unusual approach. But your case isn't normal." Dr. Jewell grew more animated as he talked. "Before offering this option, I took the liberty of calling Dr. Slimmons at Bethesda to find out more about you. He assured me you would be a super candidate for this—that you would do everything we asked during your rehabilitation."

Jack seemed intrigued by the bilateral aspect of the surgery. "Isn't that a pretty rare procedure?" he queried.

"It's never been done before at BAMC. That I know for sure. It's probably been done somewhere else, but I can't find anything in the medical literature. We would be using two separate surgical teams working independently. What do you think, Mrs. Walker?"

"Since you guys are going to be doing all the work, I'm game if you are. To paraphrase former UT football coach Darrell Royal, I'm gonna dance with the one that brung me," I replied, deciding to place my complete trust in this bright young physician.

"How does next Friday sound? That will give me time to get both teams assembled, plus the nursing support, and schedule the OR. You need to check into the hospital on Wednesday so we can do your chest X-ray, blood work, and all the other pre-op things before Friday."

Dr. Jewell then briefed us on the possible risks, complications, and expectations of such a major surgery. He emphasized that my case could be exacerbated by previous chemotherapy treatments which could lead to infection, healing problems, low platelet and white blood count, and even death.

I reported to the hospital on Wednesday with a sense of

The Fat Lady Hasn't Sung

relief, coupled with apprehension. Hopefully, I soon would be getting some diminution from the excruciating pain and be able to walk again. But to do so, I would have to sail the uncharted waters of medical history.

During afternoon rounds Dr. Jewell informed me that as a matter of policy he had placed me on the seriously ill list. He also explained that since BAMC was a teaching hospital, my history-making surgery would be witnessed by interested staff personnel and filmed for later instructional use.

Early Friday morning, with me completely nude under green sheets, a corpsman wheeled me into one of the largest OR's I had ever seen. A couple of dozen eager-faced residents and interns peered down from observation windows above the table in the middle of the room. It was like the operating amphitheaters I had seen in the movies. Even though I was a bit groggy from my pre-anesthesia medication, I looked around at the masked surgical teams and the crowd of spectators looking down from above and quipped: "If I had known I was going to have a captive audience like this, I would have dressed for the occasion."

Chapter Twenty-Five

When I awoke in the recovery room, the only sensation of discomfort I felt initially was a full bladder.

The recovery staff didn't seem to be scurrying around at the usual frenetic pace I remembered from Bethesda. After looking around a bit more I discovered why. I was the only patient at that time.

As soon as I regained my bearings sufficiently, I asked the nearest attendant for a bedpan. Almost immediately she produced a "fracture" pan—a low, nearly flat, bedpan designed to slip easily under orthopedic patients. As slim-line as the pan was, with my two sore hips, I felt like I was perched atop a mountain.

After several minutes, I realized I was not going to have success. Perhaps later, I thought, as a corpsman removed the empty pan. My discomfort would have to continue for a while longer.

It was during this first attempt to relieve my bladder that I noticed a strange, trapezoid-shaped "box" strapped between my legs. The parallel sides of the box hit me at mid-thigh and mid-calf, respectively, while the non-parallel sides traced the path of my legs and maintained a constant spread of about 30 inches at my feet. Velcro straps held the device securely in place. As I was to find out afterward, this box was to become part of my existence for quite a while.

About 45 minutes later the recovery-room head nurse, a raven-haired Army major, approached my bed with the fracture pan. "Mrs. Walker, we need to have you try to void again. If you can't go this time, we'll have to catheterize you."

That seemed to me like sufficient incentive to have success as I eased back onto the pan. Even though I had the urge and motivation, after a few minutes I knew this wasn't working.

"Have we gone yet, Mrs. Walker?" the major inquired when she returned several minutes later.

"I don't know about you, but I've come up dry," I joked as she removed the pan. "But I've got to go so bad my teeth are floating."

She ordered a catheter kit and began stripping away its plastic protective packaging as an assistant threw back my covers. When she spied the target area, she gasped in astonishment: "Oh, my! This is going to be a challenge. The area is swollen to twice the normal size!"

For the next 30 minutes the major and all of her female assistants tried unsuccessfully to find the path to my relief. Although my discomfort was becoming more intense by the minute, I tried to encourage my rescuers. "I know I'm a 'hard hit' as far as my veins are concerned, but I didn't know you'd have trouble hitting the bull's-eye there," I quipped.

Finally, with perspiration beaded on her forehead, the head nurse withdrew from her chore. "None of us seem to have the knack. Would you mind if Sgt. Barker tries? He's really quite good at this."

"I don't care if the janitor has a go at it as long as I get some relief."

Sgt. Barker gave it his best shot for about ten minutes, with plenty of supervision from his female co-workers. Realizing her expert wasn't getting the job done either, the head nurse loudly instructed someone to run and get a pediatric nurse.

When the pediatric nurse arrived, she took one look at my distended abdomen and said that if she couldn't install the catheter, she would insert a needle through my belly into my bladder and withdraw the urine that way.

Fortunately, we were able to avoid the needle method because she located the right spot after only a couple of misfires. When she inserted the catheter, I immediately felt soothing relief! In this case, "relief" was spelled by a single letter—"P."

With my discomfort assuaged, I must have drifted back to sleep because the next voice I heard sometime later was Dr. Jewell's.

"I understand you've already caused lots of excitement around here, Mrs. Walker."

I partially opened my left eye and saw Dr. Jewell standing at the side of the bed. Although he wasn't exactly smiling, he had a pleased look on his face. "How did the surgery go?" I asked earnestly.

"Pretty much according to plan. Because of the small size of your femoral shaft, it was impossible to insert a long-stemmed prosthesis. But we used a standard-stem device and lots of glue. We also had to use ten units of whole blood to replace your blood loss." Dr. Jewell busied himself as he talked, checking drains coming out of both hips.

"I thought we were going to have to call for your help during the catheter incident," I smiled.

"It's just as well you didn't. There are two procedures I haven't done since med school. And that's one of them."

"I've never had that trouble before. What caused it this time?" I wondered.

"I suspect your prior radiation, combined with the bilateral surgery, just caused more swelling than we normally see. In any case, the surgery is successfully behind us. Now it's up to you to help us get you on the road to recovery."

There was no way I could know at that moment what potholes lay along that route.

For the moment, though, I was thrilled that Dr. Jewell had

allowed Jack in the recovery room to visit with me for a few minutes. Even though he already had talked to Dr. Jewell about the surgery, I could sense Jack's relief as he embraced me and reassured me of his love.

I continued to receive superb care from the recovery room staff. Later on Friday one other patient—his head heavily bandaged following brain surgery—was wheeled in. Just by chance I had met the neurosurgeon who performed the surgery a few minutes before my own operation. I thought at the time he was a young-looking doctor. When I saw him again in recovery, attending to his patient after twelve hours of performing brain surgery, he looked as if he had aged 30 years. I don't know which is worse, being on the giving or receiving end of medicine.

A few more patients, apparently emergency cases, arrived during the night and on Saturday. But as soon as they awakened from anesthesia or became stabilized, they were sent on to a ward.

Dr. Jewell's master plan was now becoming more apparent. Even the odd day he had chosen for the surgery—Friday—started to make sense. He wanted me to spend the most critical post-surgical hours in a half-empty recovery room where I would receive the undivided care and attention of the staff.

On Saturday I was allowed for the first time to drink clear fluids, which I was able to tolerate. But when I tried my first solid food on Sunday, it seemed to trigger the kind of gastrointestinal distress I had experienced the previous year with my blockages. Dr. Jewell quickly determined that I had developed what he called an ileus, which, translated, meant a lazy intestine.

A few minutes later, Dr. Jewell approached my bed with some familiar medical equipment. "Mrs. Walker, we're going to have to insert an NG tube to suction off some of your stomach secretions. Remember when I said there were two procedures I hadn't done since med school? This is the other one."

I dreaded the thought of another NG tube, but I realized it would at least ease my stomach discomfort. "That's okay, Dr. Jewell. I've had more than my share of experience with those things. I can talk you through it."

Either my expert instructions were on target or Dr. Jewell remembered more of his medical training than he thought because he inserted the tube without too much difficulty, and I was soon getting relief.

After spending the weekend in recovery, I was ready Monday morning to return to the ward. Dr. Jewell told me earlier that he had obtained a special bed for me from the world-famous BAMC burn ward. But he hadn't prepared me adequately for the high-tech bed I saw near the nurses' station as the staff wheeled me into the ward. I was overwhelmed, and my eyes practically popped out of my head. The bed—called a circle electric—was on a round frame, like a small Ferris wheel. The big advantage of this bed was that it afforded a patient the opportunity to rotate it around so that the occupant could be in a standing position while still in bed. Then, when the time was right, one could walk directly off the bed onto the floor without having to bend the legs or body to get out of bed.

Seeing my new bed reactivated my latent Peter Pan mentality—my definition of an adult who always resisted growing up—and reminded me of my carefree childhood days riding on the Ferris wheel at Arnold's Park on Lake Okoboji, Iowa.

But I was quickly jarred back to the reality of the present as the head nurse, who had assembled the entire staff for my return, briefed her subordinates. She warned them to be extremely careful when turning, bathing, dressing, or having me use the bedpan because if something was done wrong and my hips slipped out of their sockets, I would never be able to walk again. Dr. Jewell already had warned me to be very cautious with the trapezoid-shaped frame because my legs had to be kept a certain distance apart and my hips at a specific angle to prevent dislocation.

On Tuesday—my fourth postoperative day—my lazy intestine apparently awoke because I finally had a slight feeling of hunger. Dr. Jewell immediately removed the NG tube, and I ate my first real meal in several days. Gratefully, I had no trouble keeping it down.

Dr. Jewell's normally busy schedule intensified during this

time since he also became acting head of the orthopedic clinic. Often his evening rounds were as late as 7 p.m., long after most of the other doctors had gone home. After seeing me first and then completing his rounds on the ward, he had to pass by my bed again on the way out. Each evening I said farewell in the same way: "Good night, Dr. Jewell. Have a nice evening!"

On the first couple of occasions, Dr. Jewell gave no sign of acknowledgment that I had said anything. He just kept walking, looking straight ahead. But on the third night, after I shouted my usual good-by, I saw his cupped hand come up over the back of his right shoulder and wave slightly, without turning his body or head around or uttering a sound. For the first time, he revealed an ever-so-slight chink in the traditional doctor-patient-relationship. That was as close as he came to what I thought he considered as fraternization with the patients for the rest of my stay in the hospital.

Also on Tuesday Dr. Jewell rotated my bed so that my body was vertical, and I was in a standing position. Amazingly, there was no pain—even after standing several minutes. But of course I wasn't moving anything either. The real test would come when I took my first step.

I didn't have to wait long. The next day—five days after surgery—was "W" (walk) day.

At high noon, just as in the movie, came my big performance. Dr. Jewell gathered an entourage of key members of the medical, nursing, and physical therapy staffs in case I needed help. Of course, Jack also was there to provide moral support.

Promptly at the designated time, Dr. Jewell rotated my bed so I was in a standing position again as almost a dozen pairs of eyes watched every movement. Needless to say, I was extremely nervous as he set up a walker in front of me.

"Okay, Mrs. Walker, let's see if you can walk," Dr. Jewell's voice broke the silence.

I placed my hands on the walker and shifted part of my weight off my hips. I then slowly but resolutely moved my left leg forward, followed steadily by my right. Dr. Jewell was right. My legs were the same length again. After I had walked about six feet, my audience erupted with cheers and applause. In response, I couldn't resist paraphrasing Neal Armstrong: "One small step for me. One big step for Charnley hips!"

Miraculously, there was absolutely no pain! I couldn't believe that I felt so good! A smile of joy even ventured across Dr. Jewell's face, while Jack and all the medical personnel were ecstatic. Although I must have covered about 60 or 70 feet during my first outing, I wasn't really tired. Even though Dr. Jewell told me earlier that hip replacement wasn't a magical cure, it seemed as close to magic as I was likely to see.

On the sixth post-operative day I progressed to crutches, using a four-point gait to minimize the amount of weight on my hips at any one time. I couldn't believe I could walk on crutches without pain! I knew then it was just a matter of time and rehabilitation until I would be able to walk again without assistance!

From the outset of my hospitalization, I got a lot of razzing and teasing about being a Navy wife and coming to the "first service"—the Army—for decent care. Several days after my surgery, I met a Navy corpsman who was in training at the Army's Academy of Health Science. When I told him about the ribbing I was getting, he said he would get me something I could use as an equalizer.

The next day he showed up with four or five bumper stickers bearing Navy recruiting slogans such as "Sailors Have More Fun," "Not Just a Job—An Adventure," "Join the Navy and See the World," and "Fly Navy." At my insistence, Jack attached the stickers to the crossbars of my bed. Thereafter, when the doctors made their rounds, they really laughed and thought it was a big joke that I had gone to that effort to tell my Army hosts how great the Navy was. I guess at that time they realized I was a pretty easy-going person with a relatively decent sense of humor.

Ever since my first day out of surgery I had been doing isometric exercises in bed to tighten up my muscles in anticipation of the physical therapy to follow. That time arrived on my seventh post-operative day. I was wheeled down into the basement to the PT clinic in a rigid, inclined chair which prevented my body from making a 90-degree angle with my legs—another precaution to avoid dislocating my hips.

For the next two weeks—for two sessions a day—I spent most of my time in PT trying to reeducate my muscles that they could move up and down again as well as sideways. All the exercises were designed to strengthen the muscles that held the new heads of my femurs tight and firm in their sockets so there would be no chance of my hip joints dislocating.

Those sessions in PT were sheer agony. As Jim Brady, former President Reagan's first press secretary, said years later, those people are "physical terrorists." They showed empathy but were unyielding in their quest to make patients able to walk again and return them to as normal a life as possible.

As I had done since the first days of my illness, I drew my strength and will to battle back from Jack's unswerving love and devotion. Beethoven must have had someone like him in mind for the title character in his opera *Fidelio*.

Mom and Dad arrived during this time to spend the rest of the summer with us until I could get back on my feet and operate my household on my own. Watching me agonize in PT twice a day, while visiting me at the hospital, probably wasn't much of a vacation for them either.

During these sessions I learned that one of the criteria for being released from the hospital was the ability to walk, either under one's own steam or with crutches, from the PT clinic back to the ward. This involved walking about 200 feet up a rather steep ramp to the elevator, riding the elevator to the third floor, and then walking another 200 feet to the back of the building to the female orthopedic ward.

I achieved that goal with my crutches during the last few days of July, and I knew then my stay in the hospital was about over. However, Dr. Jewell wanted me to stay until my chemotherapy could be resumed. By July 28 my blood count had reached an acceptable level, and Dr. Deas came up to my ward to inject me with my first chemotherapy at BAMC. In anticipation of my treatment, I was moved away from the nurses' station so I would have more privacy and wouldn't disturb other patients. I also transferred into a regular hospital bed.

Moving from Bethesda to BAMC didn't change the effects of the Adriamycin. Thirty minutes after Dr. Deas withdrew his syringe, I began eight hours of vomiting.

On July 30—21 days after checking into the hospital—I was released, free of hip pain but sore of muscle.

Our bedroom at home looked like it had been converted into a fitness center. Dad had rented monkey bars and other physical therapy equipment so I could continue my twice-daily sessions without having to make so many trips to the hospital. So that I could have our large bed all to myself, Jack had placed a twin-sized bed in a corner for himself.

I still had to use the trapezoid-shaped box between my legs while I was in bed. Of course, the box made it impossible for me to turn at night without help. When I needed to turn, I awakened Jack, and he had to turn me and my box as a unit. During these turns I felt like the Tin Man in "The Wizard of Oz," rusty and stiff.

Since my surgery I had been wearing long, anti-embolism stockings at all times to help prevent blood clots. They were white, full-length and went from toe to groin. Dr. Jewell wanted me to continue to wear them for another month after I left the hospital.

After Jack started his teaching job on the first of August, I spent my days exercising and walking with crutches around the block in our neighborhood a couple of times a day. Since it was a typically hot Texas August, I wore shorts over the stockings during the walks. I must have been quite a spectacle, crutching in those long, white elastic stockings. By the time I returned home, the socks had started to sag. I must have looked like "Pippy Long Stockings" in my garb.

But I didn't care. At least I was free of pain, and I knew I'd be walking on my own again soon.

CHAPTER TWENTY-SIX

As I waited in the orthopedic clinic to see Dr. Jewell for my four-week post-operative checkup, I noticed a copy of a letter filed in my health record. It was addressed to Dr. Lokey at Bethesda. It read as follows:

28 July 1975

Dear Dr. Lokey:
    This is just a brief note to let you know that Mary Walker has been able to successfully undergo a bilateral total hip replacement, so far without complication, and today started on another course of Adriamycin, Vincristine, and Procarbazine.
    The patient and her husband are a delight, and we have enjoyed dealing with them very much.

Sincerely yours,
Robert P. Witherspoon, M.D.
Major, MC
Asst. Chief, Oncology Service

Although I didn't know Dr. Witherspoon well, I recognized his name as Dr. Deas' superior in the chain of command. I was delighted my new Army doctors had taken the time and shown the thoughtfulness to keep Dr. Lokey informed of my progress.

When I crutched into Dr. Jewell's office, he was pleased with my improvement. He asked me to walk about 15 yards without crutches or cane. And he said I could start to walk around my home with just a cane. For now, he preferred that I continue to use crutches outside the house for more stability. He also wanted me to increase my physical therapy activities both in the clinic and at home.

Just about the time school started for David and Amy, I reported to Dr. Deas for my second course of chemotherapy at BAMC. Surprisingly, my blood showed I had bounced back well from the surgery and the prior chemo treatment.

That old familiar bitter taste reached my mouth even before Dr. Deas withdrew his syringe. Mom and Dad then drove me home just in time before the predictable vomiting started.

Dr. Deas also ordered another bone scan now that I was pretty well recovered from my surgery. We all rejoiced to find out there wasn't any new cancer growth. It appeared that all the vomiting and discomfort from the Adriamycin was paying off.

My folks returned to Arizona just after my birthday in September, with the promise of returning at Christmas. Jean and her family had recently relocated to Round Rock, Texas (about 100 miles northeast of San Antonio). So now, both of my parents' children lived in Texas.

As odd as it seems, things were beginning to settle into a routine. Three days of chemotherapy, followed by three days of sickness, then three weeks of respite passed before another cycle started again. It was those three days of sickness that I dreaded. At times I felt as though I were sub-human.

Dr. Deas, always considerate and full of empathy for his patients, suggested a possible remedy for my nausea and vomiting. He thought I might benefit from "relaxation therapy."

As instructed, Jack and I reported to a room in the hospital off the beaten path early on the morning of my next chemotherapy treatment. We were greeted by a pleasant, middle-aged woman who wore the insignia of a lieutenant colonel, Army Nurse Corps. She explained that she was a psychiatric nurse clinician who had specialized in relaxation therapy.

She said she would try to teach me the technique of self-relaxation which would reduce tension, anxiety, nausea, vomiting, and discomfort.

Anything with that potential sounded good to me. "If you can do that, I'll be indebted to you forever," I said enthusiastically.

"Okay, shall we get started?" she asked as she motioned for me to lie down on her couch. "What kind of background sounds are relaxing for you? I have sounds of the seashore, birds in the spring, jungle noises, wind blowing in the winter, and others." She busied herself darkening the room and seating Jack in a far corner as she awaited my reply.

"I think I'll go with the sounds of the sea. I've liked that ever since my first trip to Hawaii." I looked at Jack, and he returned a knowing smile.

She started a tape with muted sounds of waves breaking near the shore. Occasionally, the cry of a water fowl could be heard in the distance. After a couple of minutes, the nurse began speaking in a soft, soothing voice. "You are relaxing. You can feel the warm winds off the ocean caress your body. You are relaxed. Relax. . ."

She continued to speak in this way for about ten minutes. Finally, when she assumed I had achieved a light trance state, she gave the post-hypnotic suggestion that after treatment I would feel sleepy and drowsy. Furthermore, I would sleep for the time needed to awaken and feel pleasantly comfortable.

I always thought I was an individual who couldn't be hypnotized—by anyone, under any circumstances. I don't think I even came close to the state she wanted me to achieve. Not that I resisted. I *wanted* to find relief from the nausea more than anyone. But I just couldn't relax to the degree necessary. I kept thinking I might be late for my chemotherapy and I might inconvenience someone.

When the nurse turned on the lights and shut off the tape, she was absolutely beaming. She was convinced that relaxation therapy was the catholicon I needed.

Shortly after receiving my Adriamycin injection a few minutes later, I soon discovered nothing had changed. Jack got me home and settled in bed just barely before the retching started.

I never saw the psychiatric nurse again, because I just couldn't bring myself around to tell her that her beloved relaxation therapy hadn't worked for me.

My recovery from hip surgery continued without complications. Dr. Jewell thought my walk was much smoother than it had been at first. But, as he pointed out to me, I was exaggerating my body movement when walking to compensate for my somewhat decreased ability to move my hips. He referred to this as a Trendlenburg gait. I always thought it resembled the famous Charlie Chaplin walk in the character of the "Little Tramp." I abandoned my crutches completely, and I used my cane only outside the house. Dr. Jewell recommended the cane more to warn the public that I wasn't exactly a normal walker than because I really needed it.

The only problem I told Dr. Jewell about was periodic episodes of pain in my left shoulder. That was the same shoulder which had been radiated with cobalt at Bethesda to kill a tumor. Dr. Jewell diagnosed the discomfort as deterioration of the humerus head—a wearing down of the radiated shoulder joint caused from extended use of crutches.

"Why don't you let me replace your shoulder? Then you'll be like the Bionic Woman," Dr. Jewell asked jokingly, making reference to a current popular television program.

"Not unless you can put in all the other bionics," I responded in the same jesting manner. "I want to be able to hold up the car while Jack changes the tire."

When I reported to the oncology clinic for my next treatment, the staff personnel had an extremely difficult time finding a suitable vein to inject the drugs. Over time, the chemotherapy had just about wiped out all the veins in my arms, wrists, and hands. Dr. Deas had earlier discussed with me the probability of having to surgically install artificial veins—taken from cows—

or a portacath in my chest at some point in the future. But I continued to resist any more surgery and urged the oncology technicians to keep trying to find the elusive veins. Those people were wonderful! One of the technicians in particular—a pretty girl with curly hair named Michelle—often worked with me up to an hour before having success.

Since I went to the oncology clinic so often, I naturally got to know quite a few of the other patients. Many of them were in dire straits. Two or three patients whom I had met were later sent to M.D. Anderson Hospital in Houston for more aggressive chemotherapy using newer experimental drugs.

Many different oncology patients came and went. Some died and others were transferred. Of all the patients I met at BAMC—and I saw quite a few—by far the most entertaining was Andy Michell.

Andy was a young soldier stationed at Fort Hood (about 140 miles from San Antonio) who was being treated at BAMC for testicular cancer. His light-brown hair, already thinned from previous chemotherapy, partially covered his scalp in strands. His once-handsome face was now gaunt from his disease. Although his prognosis was not good, his outlook was fantastic.

During this time Jack and I had read and heard about government studies using marijuana as an anti-nausea agent for cancer patients. When I mentioned this to Andy, he was overjoyed at the prospect of using marijuana legally.

Andy rode his motorcycle from Fort Hood to San Antonio for his treatment. Since he always got sick after his injection, he usually arranged for accommodations at the Army guest house until he felt up to the return trip. Andy loved Mexican food. And since San Antonio is famous for that cuisine, he often stopped for a meal at his favorite restaurant before his chemotherapy.

Each time I saw Andy, he inquired about the status of legalizing marijuana for medicinal use. Apparently, he must have decided he couldn't wait any longer.

I arrived at the clinic one afternoon for a routine finger stick prior to my scheduled treatment the next day. I just got seated when I heard Andy's muted voice calling to me from near the door. "Mary, come outside with me for a minute. I've got something for you."

When I didn't respond immediately, he came over to where I was seated and whispered. "Mary, I've got a joint for you outside. Let's smoke it. Then we won't get sick this time."

I then realized he was serious. "Andy I don't even smoke tobacco, much less something illegal."

"But this will keep you from being sick," Andy insisted.

"Maybe so. But with my luck, I'd be the first one to get caught. I'm just not interested in illegal drugs."

"Okay, Mary. You're missing out," he replied. "But I'm going to smoke it."

"That's up to you," I responded as he left the unusually busy clinic.

Andy was gone for about 30 minutes. When he returned, I was still waiting for my blood count. Obviously, he was feeling no pain as he went directly into the treatment area. Michelle apparently had immediate success in finding a vein, and Andy returned to the waiting room within about ten minutes. As was customary after his treatment, he came over to where I was and sat down. He turned toward me and whispered: "I feel great. You're going to be sorry you didn't take a smoke."

At that moment my name was called for my blood work. When I returned to where Andy was seated, I was ready to leave. As I said goodbye, I noticed he was turning a seaweed green color. "Gee, Andy, you don't look very well," I offered.

"I don't *feel* very well!" Andy hardly got the words out before his entire Mexican dinner ended up on the chemotherapy clinic floor.

During the times I saw Andy after that, he was still optimistic about his marijuana therapy working. But Michelle told me that he always lost his lunch before he got to the guest house. Marijuana, in that form at least, didn't work for Andy. But he never failed to try. The last time I saw Andy he had received a long-sought medical transfer to a hospital near his parents' home in Illinois.

Since our move to Texas, Jack had spent every spare moment—other than doing his job, looking after the kids, and helping me when I was indisposed—trying to get a lawn started. By fall there was a ten-foot-wide green strip of grass growing next to the house. Jack had sprigged the rest of the yard with St. Augustine grass cuttings at one foot intervals. But it would take the following spring's growth to even remotely begin to cover the topsoil with grass over most of the half-acre lot.

Fall weather systems brought us more rain than usual that year. Consequently, large portions of our back yard became a muddy quagmire during rainy times.

Snoopy had adjusted pretty well to her new surroundings, and she faithfully learned to wait at the back door when she needed to go outside to the bathroom. She also learned to scratch on the door when she was ready to come back in the house. During dry periods, there was no problem. But when it was muddy, Snoopy invariably went beyond the grassy strip and ended up wearing four half-inch-thick mud shoes. This wasn't normal mud. It had a high clay content and was as sticky as glue.

Naturally, someone had to wash and dry Snoopy's feet before she could return inside. This was accomplished by filling a large, low plastic pan with water, then using one's hands to wash away the mud from each paw, and finally drying each foot with a towel. After my hip surgery, I couldn't bend down far enough to do the job. And both David and Amy tried but couldn't get the feet clean.

That left Jack who usually turned out to be the "someone" to accomplish the task.

Early one fall morning, Jack was getting ready to leave for his 8 a.m. class after teaching late the night before. An overnight Texas "norther" had brought a couple inches of rain and had dropped the temperature to near freezing.

One of the kids routinely let Snoopy out the back door to do her business. When she scratched to re-enter, Jack, who was dressed in coat and tie and on his way to the car, opened the door to find a mud-covered Snoopy looking up with her sad eyes seeking entry. Not only were each of her feet buried in mud, but the sticky mess covered her back and sides where she had rolled.

That sight was too much for Jack as he let out a rare expletive. In frustration over the mud, combined with the pressures of his new job and worry over me, Jack picked up the plastic pan and slammed it down against the sidewalk. The near-frozen plastic, as brittle as bone china after setting out in the cold overnight, shattered into a hundred pieces, some of which hit Snoopy

After getting Snoopy cleaned up, Jack was still furious. "That's it! That dog's got to go! When I get home tonight I'll make the arrangements."

Both kids were in tears over the thought of losing Snoopy. But, intuitively, I remained quite calm.

When Jack called at lunch, which he did each day to see how I was doing, his mood was cheerful as usual. "How's Snoopy?" he inquired. "Was she hurt by the plastic?"

I assured him that Snoopy was fine.

When Jack got home that evening he installed a stake in the ground near the back door and attached a short chain. Henceforth, when Snoopy needed to go out in rainy weather, she could be leashed so she couldn't get off the grassy strips.

Amy asked me at bedtime if her Daddy was going to get rid of Snoopy. "Of course not, darling," I assured her. "There was really never any doubt about it."

Chapter Twenty-Seven

When I reported for my last chemotherapy treatment before Christmas, Dr. Deas announced I had reached an important milestone.

"Mary, this is your last injection of Adriamycin. You've reached the maximum tolerable dosage."

"Oh, really?" I responded. "Does that mean I'll be finished with chemotherapy?"

"Unfortunately not. Although your latest bone scans show no evidence of new lesions, we need to remain extremely vigilant."

"But if I have to continue, I sure hate to give up the drug which seems to be turning around my cancer."

Dr. Deas examined the lymph nodes in my neck as he talked. "We really don't have any choice, Mary. Total dosage is carefully calculated based on body weight. Anymore than that could be fatal. Besides, there is some recent evidence that Adriamycin toxicity is cumulative and could lead to heart problems later on."

"Do you have any other drugs in mind as a replacement?"

"Dr. McCracken and I are currently working out the details of your new regimen. There are several possibilities."

(Dr. McCracken was the new chief of oncology service whom I had met only briefly before.)

My tolerance for Adriamycin hadn't increased during the months I had taken it, because my last shot was as bad as my first.

By the time I recovered from my latest chemotherapy blitz, our inaugural Christmas living in Texas was upon us. For the first time in our marriage, we enjoyed the holidays with both Jack's parents and my parents, plus my sister and her family, and Jack's three sisters and their families. I don't know if anyone made a definitive count, but I'm sure there were over 30 of us.

The bicentennial year of 1976 was a little over two weeks old when I made my way back to the Oncology Clinic. By this time, the doctors had come up with a new recipe of chemotherapy drugs.

Dr. Deas said the new plan involved the drug Methotrexate, followed by a recovery drug named Leukovorin. In addition, a drug called Ara-C would be used.

When I heard the name Methotrexate, a flash of recognition hit me. Jack had shown me an article in the paper about Methotrexate having been used to treat Ted Kennedy, Jr., after his leg was amputated for bone cancer. For some reason, that name stuck in my mind.

"Now, Mary," Dr. Deas began, "Methotrexate is very toxic, especially in the large doses we'll be using. We literally escort you to the brink of death, then we 'rescue' you. So it's very important to take the recovery drug precisely at the set time."

"What if I couldn't take the recovery drug on schedule?" I wondered.

"Don't even think about it! It could be fatal."

The specific Methotrexate regime involved taking large doses of the drug orally, followed by Leukovorin several hours later. This routine was to be repeated for four consecutive days. Sixteen hours after that I was to receive a subcutaneous injection of Ara-C at the hospital. This cycle was to be given every other week for six treatments at which time I was scheduled for another round of Velban and Procarbazine, the two drugs I had been taking all along with the Adriamycin. The entire course would then start all over again with the Methotrexate.

My first encounter with the new drug went pretty much as predicted. I took the Methotrexate pills in the morning, and I felt pretty good for about three hours.

Then the first signs of nausea appeared. Although the drug was different, the vomiting was just as violent and disgusting as ever. I retched every 15 to 20 minutes until about 5:30 p.m., stopping just in time to take the Leukovorin.

Jack squirted a carefully pre-measured vial of the recovery drug into a glass of root beer and handed it to me precisely at 6 p.m. Within minutes, I began feeling better as the Leukovorin began to neutralize the toxic effects of the Methotrexate.

For the next three days, I followed the same routine each day. Fortunately, the vomiting always stopped in time to take the recovery drug on schedule. On the fifth day, I reported to the Oncology Clinic for my Ara-C shot. Just as I had experienced with Adriamycin, I barely had time to return home before the vomiting hit with a vengeance.

On this new schedule, I only had a little over a week to recover from the chemotherapeutic insult to my body before the whole thing started again.

Just as I had done during the first cycle, I took the Methotrexate in the morning, dreading the inevitable nausea to follow. When the vomiting started, I felt even sicker than I had remembered from before.

When Jack got home from work around 4:30, I was still retching every 15 minutes with no letup in sight. He comforted me as best he could, but both of us realized there was nothing either of us could do except wait it out.

At 5:45 Jack looked terribly worried as he emptied the pink pan again. "Mary, darlin', you've got 15 minutes before you have to take the Leukovorin. And you're still vomiting like you'll never stop."

"Oh, Jack," I moaned. "I'm so sick. I can't take the recovery drug."

Jack was horrified at what I was saying. "You've got to take it! There isn't any choice."

At five minutes before six, Jack called Dr. Deas. Luckily, he happened to be on call and was at his office. When Jack explained what was happening, Dr. Deas said to bring me in immediately.

Jack quickly rounded up the kids from playing, and helped me stump out to the car. I was so weak from vomiting all day that I really struggled to make it.

David and Amy rode in the front seat with Jack, freeing up the back seat for me and my ever-present pink pan. As I laid there in the speeding car violently vomiting every few minutes, I looked up through the rear window at the darkening Texas sky and wondered how it would all end.

When Jack pulled up to the nearest stairway to Dr. Deas' third floor office, I knew I couldn't make it. Even with normal hips, I was too weak to make it up three flights of stairs while vomiting almost constantly.

Jack bounded up the stairs four at a time and, within a couple of minutes, returned with Dr. Deas who was carrying a syringe of Leukovorin. Dr. Deas climbed into the back seat with me, wiped my arm with an alcohol swab, and injected the medicine. I vomited once more after the shot, but, within minutes, it was clear my nausea was subsiding as the recovery drug began to neutralize the Methotrexate.

Dr. Deas sat on the curb by my open door until he was sure I had finished vomiting. He assured me that although I was late taking the recovery drug, I was still within the window of safety. I have always maintained that oncologists are a special breed of physician. Without exception, all of them I've known are very empathic and are willing to take as much time as necessary to learn of any problems and allay any fears and worries.

Dr. Deas' willingness to take extraordinary measures on my behalf was more typical of the oncologists I've known than the exception.

After my adverse reaction, Dr. Deas switched the time of day

I was to take the Methotrexate. Instead of taking it in the morning, he instructed me to take it at bedtime. By going to sleep shortly after taking the pills, Dr. Deas hoped I might just sleep my nausea away for the rest of the night.

The first time I tried the new schedule, I slept until about 2 a.m. when I awoke from the nausea and immediately threw up. Vomiting continued every 20 minutes or so until around daybreak when Jack brought me the Leukovorin. This seemed to be a better schedule because more time elapsed before I got sick, and I often dozed between the nausea attacks. For the rest of the time I was on Methotrexate, I followed this schedule without ever having a repeat of the emergency shot in the back seat of the car.

I continued to have bone scans about every three months during this time to check on any new activity and to keep tabs on the older spots. We all rejoiced as each new scan showed no evidence of any new lesions and continued to show shrinkage of the old tumors.

After I had been off Adriamycin for about six weeks, I noticed some new "peach fuzz" growing on my head. The hair was as fine as a baby's. But it was hair! I was delighted that I might be able to flip my wig soon. And, as a bonus, based on the texture of the new growth, it looked like my hair might come in curly the second time around. I didn't find that too surprising since my mother had naturally-curly hair. I was so elated about the prospect of getting curly hair that I thought (in a moment of weakness) all the agony from the Adriamycin almost had been worthwhile.

As my hair came back thicker, however, it was obvious that it was still as straight as a board.

One day when I was in Dr. Deas' office for a treatment, I was sharing with him my joy about getting my hair back along with my disappointment about its lack of curliness.

Dr. Deas laughed loudly at my plight. "Well, Mary, maybe you and I can work out a transplant if you really want curly hair," he joked as he rubbed the top of his Afro haircut.

"Maybe so," I laughed. "You could easily spare some."

By now, life in our new surroundings had settled into a routine. David and Amy had adjusted well in their new school, and they seemed to be enjoying living in Texas, particularly the outdoors.

As summer neared, Jack and I decided to put in a backyard swimming pool. My orthopedic doctors kept saying that swimming was the best possible exercise for me. Also I hated to be seen at public pools. Instead of the name "scarface," I could answer to "scarleg."

Excavation for the pool began in April. But because of unusually heavy rains and the necessity to cut through almost solid rock, that phase of construction lasted almost six weeks. The workmen drilled holes into the stone, filled them with dynamite, and then blasted loose huge chunks which were then hauled away. Poor Snoopy! As soon as the blasting began, she shivered and salivated the rest of the day.

When the pool was finished in the middle of June, our backyard took on the look of a super playground. The water area was flanked by half a basketball court in one corner of the yard and a badminton area in the other. There was still another area for playing croquet.

Naturally, something that appealing caused our home and yard to become a mecca for most of the neighborhood kids.

When I wasn't taking chemotherapy, it seems most of the summer was spent life guarding and riding herd on the dozens of kids who dropped by during the day. Every couple of hours I refreshed the gathering with lemonade and snacks. Even my chemotherapy treatments didn't slow down the procession of kids. It had become almost commonplace for David and Amy's mother to be sick every three weeks or so. When I was too sick to watch the youngsters, I pressed Jack into service. He acted as lifeguard and served refreshments as I threw up in our bedroom. Every 30 minutes he checked on me and emptied my pink pan.

My strange walking gait must have shifted pressure to new areas of my feet since I developed pain in the left heel, ankle, and calf. Shortly after the big Fourth of July Bicentennial celebration,

Dr. Jewell diagnosed the problem as a stress fracture of the left heel. He suggested I immobilize my foot and immediately fitted me with an Army "designer" clog, to be worn for four to six weeks.

The next glitch in an otherwise uneventful late summer and fall came in early December. During a routine bone scan the radiologist noted some evidence of increased "uptake" on the distal ends (the ends near the knees) of both femurs. This news sent the orthopedic doctors into a tailspin (along with Jack). They speculated this could be advancing metastatic disease uncontrolled by drug therapy. The oncologists, however, remained calm and ordered more X-rays and another bone scan. After a month's deliberation, it was finally decided that this change represented more thinning of the radiated bone rather than new cancer activity.

Another bone scan in early 1977 yielded extremely positive news. There were no new lesions, and all the original inoperable tumors essentially were gone. It was clear that chemotherapy had done its job!

This was the weapon I needed to start fighting the oncologists about going off of chemotherapy. I pointed out to Dr. Deas that I now had been on chemotherapy for three years—much longer than anyone I had heard of or read about.

But Dr. Deas was quite satisfied with the status quo. He didn't want to take any risks since I was doing so well. Consequently, my first attempt was unsuccessful.

By March I was more insistent as I visited with Dr. Deas prior to another treatment. "Dr. Deas, we've got to bite the bullet. I can't live the rest of my life on chemotherapy. You've got to take me off."

"I know, Mary. It's just that I don't want to do anything to upset the apple cart when you're doing so well. Disease involving bone is relatively difficult to evaluate. That's because the presence or absence of findings on bone scans frequently may not be indicative of the true status of your disease."

"You don't think I have any active disease, do you?"

"No, I don't. I actually think your disease has been stable

since you arrived here."

"Well, there. The chemotherapy worked. You can' keep me on this stuff forever. It's an unreal life."

My persistence seemed to have swung Dr. Deas a bit my way. He ordered another bone scan for the end of March, along with X-rays and blood tests, and agreed to present my case at an oncology staff meeting in April.

Although Dr. Deas had yielded somewhat, Jack was still extremely reluctant to do anything which could possibly reverse my recovery. Although I used the same arguments with him as I had with Dr. Deas, he remained very apprehensive about me stopping chemotherapy at this time.

From a practical point of view, my veins had deteriorated so badly that I either had to stop chemotherapy or have an artificial vein put in.

During my next treatment in April, Dr. Deas said he had presented my case to the staff, and some decision would be forthcoming in May.

When Jack and I walked into his office in May, Dr. Deas' face was radiant with happiness. "I've got good news! You won't have any more chemotherapy treatments!"

I was so happy I was speechless for one of the few times in my life.

When I finally found words to reply, I could only say "Thank you, Dr. Deas! Thank you!"

But Dr. Deas also had some very precise conditions. "We're going to watch you *very* carefully. We want you to come in for a check every 30 days for the next six months. We need bone scans every two months. We want you to keep a close eye on your body and be aware of any changes. If there is *any* change, come in immediately."

I was so happy to be getting off chemotherapy that I would have agreed to almost any conditions.

Dr. Deas also informed us that he was being transferred to El Paso. A new oncologist, Dr. Shildt, would be following me in the future. Since this was the last time we would see each other, Dr.

Deas asked Jack if he could give me a goodbye kiss.

"You bet," Jack agreed. "We're so grateful for everything you've done, *I'd* kiss you if the Army wouldn't court martial you," he quipped.

Dr. Deas gave me a hug and kissed me on the cheek. "Goodbye, Mary. Keep on fighting. God bless you!"

When Jack and I left the clinic, I was euphoric. After over three years, I was *finally* off of chemotherapy! I now could look forward to summer and hopefully the prospect of a reasonably normal life. Although Jack didn't want to spoil my joy, I could tell that he was very apprehensive about stopping the drugs, fearful that the cancer could become active again.

When we got home I told Jack I'd like to call Dr. Lokey to share the good news.

After numerous attempts to find him in Atlanta, I finally got through to his office and heard a man's voice speaking in a soft, Southern accent.

"Dr. Lokey?"

"Yes."

"I don't know if you remember me or not. I'm Mary Walker."

"Oh, yes. I know exactly who you are."

"Dr. Lokey, I know you'll be overjoyed to learn that my cancer is in remission, and, as of today, I'm off of chemotherapy!"

Dr. Lokey was silent for a moment, apparently very moved. "I'm so happy for you, Mary. You made my day. I'm anxious to tell my patients about you—my first success story!"

When I hung up the phone, I sat there for a few minutes trying to absorb the magnitude of what we had accomplished. Jack came over and embraced me for a long, silent hug.

I felt such a warm glow knowing that—at least for now—I had beaten the odds.

Chapter Twenty-Eight

I had to pinch myself several times during May to make sure I wasn't dreaming. Finally, after more than three years of enduring the most agonizing sickness and pain imaginable, I was now off of chemotherapy!

The drugs had saved my life. But at the same time, they almost killed me.

My first treatment caused severe internal bleeding which would have meant certain death without divine intervention and the skills of a dedicated surgeon. Every treatment caused hours of gut-wrenching nausea and vomiting. My body was as dehydrated as the Mojave Desert and ached like I had been run over by a steam roller. The hair on my head fell out by the handful; eventually, I even lost my eyebrows and eyelashes. My pallor turned grey, my face became gaunt, and my body, skeleton-like.

Would I go through it all over again?

Absolutely! Without any doubts!

Why? That question has been posed to me probably more than any other.

The answer is simple: I chose life! By the time my cancer was diagnosed, it was inoperable. Chemotherapy was my *only* hope. So I decided I would have to go with the only means available, and I would be successful.

I felt as emphatic about my ultimate success as Calaf does at the end of his brilliant aria, "*Nesun Dorma,*" in Puccini's *Turandot* where he sings "*Vincerò!* [I shall conquer!]"

On the Saturday after Dr. Deas gave us the good news, Jack wanted to go shopping. Since Jack hates to shop, I knew this must be special. When he drove the four of us to the local Cadillac dealership, I thought the strain of the past three and half years had finally gotten to him.

Jack led us inside the showroom directly to a white Sedan de Ville with red leather seats and matching interior trim. "Well, how do you like it?" Jack asked as the kids scampered into the back seat voicing their approbation.

"Are you out of your mind, Jack? We can't afford this," I responded in shock.

"We can't afford not to have it. It's really more economical than buying a stripped down economy car and then having to add on the extras."

"But it's so ostentatious. We've always owned Chevrolets."

"Look, Mary, it's a safe, comfortable car. So what if it also happens to be luxurious. I think you deserve a little luxury."

The more we talked, the more I could visualize that feeling of well being driving a car like that provided.

A salesman gave us the keys to a similarly-equipped car and suggested we take it for a drive. That proved to be the clincher. After that, even I couldn't resist any longer.

As part of our continuing celebration of the end of my chemotherapy, we decided to drive our new car to Arizona during the summer to see my parents. While we were there, we all went up to the Grand Canyon. For me, the Grand Canyon is a spectacle of awesome grandeur and natural history significance unequaled anywhere on earth.

For the rest of the summer and fall, my radiated left shoulder got progressively worse. Since I am left-handed, routine household tasks such as ironing and cleaning—even writing—became very painful.

In November, I reluctantly returned to the Orthopedic Clinic to try to find some relief. By now, Dr. Jewell had been separated from the Army to pursue a civilian practice somewhere back east. When my name was called, I carried my new X-rays and followed a familiar-looking doctor back to his examining room where he introduced himself as Dr. McIlwain. It was then that I placed name and face together. He was one of the orthopedic residents who made rounds each day with Dr. Jewell during my hip replacements.

Dr. McIlwain positioned my X-rays on his viewer and began studying them closely. While he looked at the images, my mind wandered back to the first time I ever saw him.

Mom and Dad were visiting me at the hospital on a Saturday morning while I was recuperating from my hip surgery.

In military hospitals, since doctors not on duty are technically off on weekends, rounds are often made later in the day on Saturday and Sunday and in civilian clothes.

On that Saturday the doctors were making their rounds around mid-morning, after the start of visiting hours. In addition to my parents, there were quite a few other visitors on the ward as well.

As the three of us were talking, my mother noticed a young man dressed in blue jeans and a knit shirt visiting with an older lady located diagonally across the ward.

"Isn't that nice?" my mother asked, interrupting our conversation. "That lady's grandson has come to visit her while she's here in the hospital."

"Mother," I whispered, almost breaking up with laughter, "that's not her grandson. That's her doctor!"

My mother was shocked that anyone who looked so young could be a doctor. That young-looking doctor, it turned out, was Dr. McIlwain.

As I looked at him examining my X-rays, I thought he hadn't aged much since I last saw him. He still had the same boyish good looks and quick smile.

"Well, Mrs. Walker," Dr. McIlwain began, still looking at the X-rays, "I can understand why you're having pain in your shoulder. The head of your humerus looks like the moon's surface. It's all pock-marked and filled with craters."

"Gosh, I didn't realize it had deteriorated that much since Dr. Jewell last saw it. Do you think using crutches caused all that damage?"

"That, plus we're dealing with radiated bone," Dr. McIlwain speculated. "In spite of the way it looks, I think we should try something conservative."

"What do you have in mind?"

"Let's try a cortisone shot. Then come back in a month, and we'll follow up with another."

Dr. McIlwain inserted a long needle all the way into the joint bone and slowly discharged the cortisone into the area, moving the needle from time to time to get complete coverage. After the initial sharp pain of the needle, the normal shoulder discomfort seemed to ease up a bit. I was cautiously optimistic when I left the clinic that this conservative treatment just might be the cure to my shoulder pain.

I was a little disheartened, however, when I reported back a month later. Either the cortisone had not become fully activated, or it wasn't doing the job.

I told Dr. McIlwain my shoulder wasn't any better, and it might be a bit worse.

"I was going to give you a second cortisone shot. But from what you've told me, it doesn't seem to be helping at all." Dr. McIlwain moved my shoulder as he talked. "I'm very reluctant to put any more steroids in you when they're not helping."

"Is there any other shot you can use?"

"Not really. The only real relief is to have your shoulder replaced. But let me quickly add that is very serious surgery and not something to take lightly."

My thoughts went back to Dr. Jewell when he joked about making me into the Bionic Woman. And now Dr. McIlwain may end up with that dubious honor.

"Talk it over with your husband, Mrs. Walker. If you both concur, then we'll go ahead and schedule the surgery. Since you're not on crutches anymore—and your shoulder really is not a weight-bearing joint—you should do quite well."

Not surprisingly, Jack wasn't too keen on me having more surgery. He wanted to be sure that that was the only alternative. When I assured him my choice was shoulder replacement or living with constant pain, he reluctantly agreed.

I scheduled the surgery for early January since I knew Mom and Dad were going to be with us for the Christmas holidays, and I knew they would stay on to help out for awhile during and after my surgery.

Meanwhile, shortly after New Year's Day of 1978, Jack's dad became ill and checked into a civilian hospital. John Walker had a dry, English sense of humor, and his manner of speaking reminded me of the late character actor, Walter Brennan. He and I always enjoyed a good relationship, and I was the only child or spouse of a child who could tease him with impunity.

Jack and I visited his dad on Sunday before I was to check into BAMC on Monday. When we entered his hospital room, he was sitting up eating his dinner.

After a nice visit, I kissed him goodbye as Jack and I prepared to leave. "I check into the hospital tomorrow to get a new shoulder," I told him. "Both of us probably will be released about the same time. Then we'll celebrate!"

Jack's dad nodded in agreement as he wished me good luck during my surgery and said farewell.

I checked into the hospital early the next morning to begin my pre-operation tests. As I made my rounds, I thought how different this surgery was going to be compared to all the others I had had since 1974. For the first time in four years I would be able to get up and walk around like a normal person during my recuperation.

During afternoon rounds, Dr. McIlwain informed me that all my pre-op tests were back and were within normal limits. He also said that Dr. Nelson, chief of orthopedics, wanted to talk to me after dinner.

At 7 p.m. I made my way to the orthopedic office. As I entered the room, Dr. Nelson, a large, grey-haired man, rose to his feet. Dr. McIlwain was standing to one side.

"Thanks for coming by, Mrs. Walker," Dr. Nelson began. "I wanted to talk to you personally to let you know just how serious shoulder replacement is."

I nodded my understanding as he continued. "We haven't done many of these before here at BAMC. This surgery certainly is not in the tried-and-true category of hip replacement."

"But it's not experimental, is it?" I asked.

"No, but we just haven't had much experience with it," Dr. Nelson added. "I'm sure Dr. McIlwain had told you that we will have to excise or cut off your humeral head and insert a Neer prosthetic replacement."

"I don't think he mentioned Neer. Let me guess though. That must be named for Dr. Neer," I added. By now I had become pretty familiar with some of the orthopedic pioneers. The doctors remained silent as I continued. "What I'd like to know is whether or not this surgery could make me a whole lot better and not any worse."

Both doctors agreed it could.

"In that case, I'm ready if you are," I added.

When I returned to the ward, a nurse gave me a betadine kit—containing a red, iodine type soap—with instructions to scrub the area of the incision-to-be at least twice that night and once the next morning. After the morning scrub, I was told to leave the soap on to dry. That always made my skin feel tight and stretched like animal hides on an Indian teepee.

As I scrubbed away on my shoulder, I thought about my long association with betadine solution and my introduction to it in Bremerhaven, Germany.

On a cold spring morning in 1963 I was getting ready to go to a bridge luncheon. I was running a bit late as I tried to get something organized for Jack's lunch. I took out a package of frozen hamburger patties so they could thaw somewhat while I finished washing my hair. When I returned to the kitchen, the six patties were still firmly frozen together. Since I was unsuccessful in prying them apart with a table knife, I decided to try my sharpest paring knife to expedite the job.

Initially, I held the frozen meat against my abdomen with one hand and used the knife in the other like an ice pick to stab the patties and break them apart. I couldn't get enough leverage that way, so I grasped the patties with my right hand and held them out in front of me, using the knife to stick the meat. I drew back and gave a mighty plunge into the burgers. When the sharp knife point hit the frozen mass, it deflected off the patties, burying itself in my right palm, between the thumb and forefinger.

Initially, the only thing I felt was a sensation similar to an electric shock. But when I looked down, I saw at least an inch of knife blade sticking out through the back of my hand. The knife had gone right through my hand!

I thought to myself, "Oh, my Lord! Now look what I've done!" Without thinking about possible consequences, I quickly pulled the knife back out, setting off the same electrical shock sensation I had felt moments before.

Extracting the knife blade was like pulling the plug on a high-pressure container. Blood squirted everywhere! Within seconds, my kitchen was a blood-spattered eyesore.

I grabbed the kitchen towel and wrapped it around my hand. My main concern at that point was the terrible mess I was making. Oddly enough, there wasn't much pain. I guess holding the frozen meat had partially anesthetized my hand.

Within a short time I bled through the kitchen towel, so I went to the bathroom and wrapped a couple of bath towels tightly around the bloody mess.

I finally began to realize that I needed to go to the hospital for stitches. Now I'm really going to be late for bridge, I thought. And I wasn't even dressed yet.

But how would I get to the hospital? I knew I couldn't drive our stick-shift Volkswagen myself with my right hand wrapped to the size of a football. I'd have to find someone to drive me.

I ran up and down our stairwell, knocking on every door, only to find no one at home. After giving up on my nearest neighbors, I looked out our door and saw Doris Ford, who lived on the third floor of the next stairwell, just entering the front door of the building.

I dashed over to her entrance, bounded up the three flights of stairs, and knocked on her door. She gasped when she saw the blood-soaked towels.

"Doris, I really need your help," I explained. "I ran a knife through my hand, and I must get to the hospital as soon as possible. Would you drive me in my car?"

"Oh, Mary, I wish I could. But I never learned how to drive a car with a clutch," Doris responded with a slight tinge of embarrassment.

"Could you take me in your car then?"

"Mary, you're bleeding so badly. Bob and I just got a brand new Mercedes. I'd die if any blood got on the carpet or seats," Doris explained, still staring at the bloody towels.

"Look, Doris, I'm getting desperate. I promise I'll hold my hand out the window so I can't drip inside if you'll just drive me to the hospital."

Doris looked at me with an air of discomfiture. "How foolish of me. Of course I'll drive you, Mary. I'll meet you in five minutes."

I ran back to our apartment and changed towels. All my running up and down stairs had kept the blood pumping from the wound.

Doris was already waiting at my stairwell door in her cream-colored limousine when I came out of the building.

True to my word, I held my hand out the window all the way to the hospital even though it was a cold day. I was not going to be responsible for getting blood on her car's champagne interior.

At the hospital, the emergency room doctor seemed irritated by my predicament. "You would have been better off leaving the knife in your hand," he scolded as he cleaned up the wound. By now the bleeding had slowed down. "By pulling it out, you've cut nerves at least, and you may have severed tendons and ligaments."

Since I had no defense for my stupid actions, I remained quiet and listened.

"There's no way to sew up a puncture wound like this. I want you to soak your hand four times a day in betadine solution." The doctor continued chastising me as he applied a sterile bandage. "And you better hope and pray it heals from inside out without getting infected. That knife had to be contaminated with bacteria."

Before I left the emergency room, the doctor gave me a tetanus shot and prescriptions for antibiotic and pain medications.

When I returned home, our apartment looked like a scene from the movie *Psycho*. Blood was spattered on the walls, floor, and counters. I cleaned up some of the worst of the mess, but I needed Jack's help to finish the job. Besides, there was still time to join the bridge game if I hurried. After calling one of the players, she picked me up on her way to the club.

When Jack came home and saw the bloody room, he was frantic. Every imaginable scenario of what could have happened to me raced through his mind. When he reached me by phone at the club, his fear turned to exasperation as I told him about my careless accident. Later that day, he broke off the sharp tips on all my kitchen knives.

Jack and I had made plans weeks earlier to drive to Copenhagen during the approaching weekend. But since my knife accident occurred on Thursday, Jack suggested cancelling our hotel reservation and postponing our trip.

"Why?" I asked. "I can soak my hand in Copenhagen and while coming and going as well as I can here. Besides, the trip will help get my mind off my injury."

I must have convinced Jack, because shortly after noon the next day we were en route to Copenhagen. We drove to Hamburg, then to Flensburg at the northern tip of Germany, and then crossed the border into Denmark. From there we traveled to the Danish cities of Kolding, Odense, and Nyborg where we boarded a car ferry to make the hour and 40 minute passage across the Kattegat of the Baltic Sea.

After parking our car on the ship, we headed directly for the dining room where we had made dinner reservations. Dining at sea was a pleasure both of us shared. In addition to a delightful way to pass the time, this would give me an opportunity to soak my hand for the third time that day.

Our waiter, stiff and proper in his formal attire, showed us the menu. While we were making our selections, I asked the waiter if he would fill a stainless steel pan (which I had carried with me) with warm water. He obsequiously agreed and hurried off to fetch the water.

He returned quickly and took our orders. After he sped off to the kitchen, I discreetly placed the pan on the cushion between me and the bulkhead. I then poured in the designated amount of the red betadine solution, mixed it around in the water, and began soaking my hand.

When our waiter returned with our food, his normal chalky pallor quickly turned into a bilious green when he saw my hand in the red water. He literally threw down our food on the table and beat a hasty retreat. I remember thinking it was rather odd for a sea-going person to get sea-sick on such calm waters.

Our waiter never returned during the meal. When we were ready to order coffee, Jack summoned the head waiter and asked what had happened to our server. (My napkin now was discreetly covering my hand and the pan.)

"Regrettably, he's indisposed," the head waiter replied in impeccable English. "He gets deathly ill at the sight of blood. But I can't imagine where he could have seen blood on this ship."

When we debarked at Korsor and began driving the remaining short distance to Copenhagen, we were still laughing at what that waiter must have thought that pan of betadine solution was.

Miraculously, the knife wound healed without getting infected. However, the emergency room doctor was right. I had cut a major nerve since I lost all feeling in my fore- and middle fingers.

Several months later, since the Bremerhaven Army Hospital lacked that capability, I went to Landstuhl Army Hospital in southern Germany for surgery to reconnect my severed nerve.

Once more, betadine soap played a prominent role in my pre-op preparations.

Chapter Twenty-Nine

Early on the day of my scheduled shoulder surgery, I took another shower with betadine soap.

I finished drying off and started back toward my bed. Just as I passed the main door to the ward, Jack opened it and came in. He looked tired and upset.

"Jack, Honey, what are you doing here so early?" I asked, surprised to see him.

"Dad died a couple hours ago," he explained. "I was just taking Mom to the hospital. Unfortunately, we didn't get there in time. His doctor said it must have been a massive heart attack."

I was shocked. I had just seen Jack's dad Sunday night. He didn't seem sick enough to die. And he didn't have a history of heart disease.

"I'm so sorry, Jack. I think I'd better postpone my surgery," I offered, still unable to believe what I had just heard.

"No, there's really nothing you can do. I have to make the funeral arrangements later today. I'd really prefer you to go ahead with the surgery as planned."

"But at least I could be some moral support if I'm with you."

Although I had not yet lost either of my parents, I could empathize with him. "I just wish there was some way to help you."

He finally persuaded me that it was best to go with the original plan.

Jack accompanied me to the elevator leading to the operating room and kissed me goodbye. The last thing I recalled before the anesthesia overtook me was the haunting sadness in his eyes.

The next event I remember was back on the ward where Jack, in his customary role, was waiting. Although I'm sure I had awakened enough in the recovery room to be transferred, I couldn't remember being there.

The nursing staff was still getting me settled in my bed when Dr. McIlwain showed up in his green scrubs. He looked tired, but he smiled as he greeted me. "How're you feeling, Mary?"

"Pretty good. Just a little groggy."

"I wanted you to know that the surgery went well. Your previous cobalt treatments gave us a couple of problems, however. Some of your muscles were literally glued to your bone. We also had to remove a fairly large vein for that reason."

"Will that affect my recovery?"

"It shouldn't. The main thing is to be very careful. Right now your shoulder isn't strong enough to support the weight of your arm," Dr. McIlwain explained as he checked the drain coming from the wound. "That's why you're wearing this Jacksonville sling."

"Don't worry. I'll be careful. I don't want my arm to drop off," I said whimsically.

"If that happens, we'll just stick it back on with super glue," Dr. McIlwain kidded me back.

My left arm was resting in an olive drab-colored sling which went around my neck. Another piece of cloth encircled my upper body and held my arm tightly against my chest, making my shoulder and arm completely immobile.

Later that day I got out of bed to go to the bathroom, using the monkey bar to pull up with my right arm and swing my legs around to touch the floor. By being able to walk immediately after surgery, I was optimistic that my recovery would go well.

A couple of days later Jack's dad was buried. Even though I couldn't attend the funeral, it was a sad occasion knowing that I'd never see him again. But it was also a joy to see all of Jack's siblings once more, including brothers from both coasts of the United States.

In medical parlance, my recovery was "unremarkable"—that is, it was without complications. After twelve days Dr. McIlwain discharged me with the stern admonition not to lift anything with my left arm heavier than a fork.

The postoperative plan required me to continue wearing my Jacksonville sling and to come back to the hospital daily for physical therapy.

At my first PT session I asked the therapist if I could do some needlework while I was recuperating. I have always loved counted cross-stitch, needlepoint, and knitting.

"Fine," the therapist agreed. "It might help tune up the smaller muscles before we're ready to work on the larger ones."

"Thanks. I started knitting a baby blanket for my neighbor before my surgery. Now maybe I'll finish it before her baby graduates from high school."

My first PT routine involved the therapist removing my sling and gently assisting me to lower my arm while I bent my body so that my arm and hand hung freely like a pendulum. I then moved my arm clockwise in a small circle for about two minutes before reversing the movement in the other direction for an equal amount of time. I gradually worked up to doing about 20 minutes of these pendulum exercises four times a day.

After three weeks of the same pendulum exercises, my physical therapist announced a change. "Today we're going to start very gradually on external rotation of your shoulder—with assistance of course."

"Oh, good! I've done so many pendulum exercises I was beginning to feel like a grandfather clock," I joked.

External rotation exercises required the therapist to grasp my arm and raise it up perpendicular to my body. A few days after starting this new routine, we were doing about 20 repetitions of this exercise at each session.

My mother and father extended their visit for about a week more after I got home from the hospital. They were a tremendous help, but I felt confident I could carry on without them. After all, my legs worked well with my two artificial hips, and I could drive our car, thanks to the automatic transmission. I also had full use of my right arm and hand.

As I drove myself to physical therapy, I thought about the first time my arm was in an Army sling.

While Jack and I were in Bremerhaven, numerous visiting dignitaries came through "on business," in many cases to justify taking an expensive European vacation at government expense.

During one cold January, an admiral from Washington, D.C., determined that Jack's command would have the pleasure of his company for a couple of days. Jack's commanding officer, Captain Portabella, decided to hold a command-performance dinner-dance at the Navy Officers' Club with the admiral as guest of honor. Since this admiral was well known throughout the Navy as "Silent Hal" for his quiet personality, Captain Portabella decided to seat me on the admiral's right to help keep the conversation going during dinner.

Making small talk with anyone has always come easy for me. During the appetizer course, I tried to discuss travel. "Have you been in Europe before?" I asked him to get started on the subject.

"Yes," responded Silent Hal.

Further attempts to discuss this subject elicited similar monosyllabic responses.

During the main course, I brought up sports. "How're the Washington Redskins doing this year?"

"Okay."

"I'm a Dallas Cowboys and Houston Oilers fan myself," I continued.

"Really?"

After he uttered no more than a dozen words on sports, I thought I'd try something else during dessert. "Jack and I have enjoyed going to the opera houses of Europe," I began. "We recently saw a great performance of Verdi's *Don Carlo* in Hamburg. Boris Christoff was overwhelming in the role of Phillip II."

"Don't care much for opera myself."

By this time I was desperate. "What *is* this guy interested in," I wondered as I racked my brain for a subject which might pique some conversation.

Finally, I thought about a subject that was almost too obvious. "What about hobbies? Do you have any hobbies?"

"Why, yes. I'm a philatelist."

The word sounded familiar, but its exact meaning eluded me. I quickly did a mental check on Greek prefixes and suffixes, but I still couldn't decipher it.

Silent Hal, sensing my potential embarrassment at not knowing the word, helped me along. "Most people would just say I was a stamp collector."

From that point on, the whole evening changed. Silent Hal suddenly became "Loquacious Hal." He told me everything I ever wanted to know about stamps and stamp collecting and then some.

Jack, who had been stuck at the other end of the table, sensed that I needed some relief. When the band began playing after dinner, Jack interrupted the stamp talk and asked me to dance. We danced through several romantic tunes until the band struck up a polka. That music is always Jack's cue to sit down.

When Jack returned me to my seat, Captain Portabella gave him a dirty look for leaving the admiral stranded for several minutes during our dance. But it didn't take long for Silent Hal to pick up where he left off on his philatelical discourse.

Perhaps sensing that he might lose his captive audience to another dance partner, the admiral asked me to dance. As soon as we reached the floor, the band picked up the pace to what we used to call a "jitterbug." (I had noticed the club manager sprinkling dance floor sparkle over the surface just before our arrival).

By now, Silent Hal was really out of his shell. He not only had found an attentive listener about his hobby, but he also had a dance partner almost half his age.

His dance steps and moves were not too contemporary. In fact, he kept using a 1940's style movement of swinging me out and pulling me back toward him.

On one of those swing outs, I lost my footing on the slippery floor and landed flat on my back on the oak surface. On my way down, I tried to cushion my fall with my right arm.

The moment my body hit the floor, the orchestra stopped playing, and, for a few seconds, everyone seemed transfixed like statues as I looked up at them.

Jack was the first person to arrive and help me up. Initially, I felt more embarrassment than pain. Within a few minutes, however, I knew from the swelling and discomfort that I had injured my right wrist. Jack insisted that we go to the hospital immediately, and as I said goodnight to the admiral, he was still trying to tell me about his latest stamp auction.

When Jack and I reached the parking lot, we noticed that Michael Johns, a bachelor ensign who worked for Jack, was stuck in a snow bank, and his Alpha Romeo sports car was blocking us.

Michael apparently had been trying for some time to extricate his car since the smell of burning rubber was thick in the night air. By now his frustration level was soaring as he continued again and again to spin his tires against the hard-packed snow. Even with Jack's help pushing as Michael raced the engine, the vehicle remained stuck.

Finally, in an act of great desperation, Michael ripped off his white silk scarf from around the collar of his bridge coat and placed the cloth under his right tire for more traction. The tread of the tire grasped the scarf, spun it around, and threw it out behind his car without moving the vehicle at all.

By the time Michael tried the scarf trick a few more times, the couple parked behind us came out of the club and moved their car, thus freeing up an egress for us.

At the hospital, X-rays revealed I had suffered a dislocated wrist. A doctor put a cast on me and placed my arm in a government-issued sling. He apologized that the olive drab color didn't complement my dinner dress.

To this day, I don't know if Silent Hal found another victim that night or how Ensign Johns ever got his car out of the snow bank.

Six weeks after my shoulder surgery, the therapist started me lifting a one-pound barbell. "I want your assurance that I'm not going to end up looking like Gargantua," I wisecracked as he assisted me initially in lifting the weight.

"For sure, not Gargantua. But I can't guarantee you won't have some Amazon traits," he responded in kind.

Eventually, I progressed to using a five-pound barbell. By early summer I had regained full use of my left arm and shoulder. And, gratefully, I didn't end up looking like Gargantua or an Amazon.

Chapter Thirty

With three of my major joints now artificial, I was in a good position to lay claim to the title of the Bionic Woman.

Even though I couldn't hold up the car to change a flat tire, I was at least free of much of the pain and discomfort I had experienced since 1973.

When I look at the long scars over both my hips and see the crimson cut on my left shoulder, I don't see disfigurement. I also don't feel bitter. Instead, I rejoice that I was born at a time when the wonders of modern medicine are available. Had I entered life 20 years earlier, it is doubtful that I would be alive, much less be able to walk and to have the use of both arms.

During the rest of 1978 I continued my shoulder exercises. By now, the five-pound barbell was as easy to lift as the one-pound weight was earlier in my rehabilitation. The best news of all was that my regular oncology and orthopedic checkups and scans continued to be good.

One of the joys of living in Texas is being able to be outdoors most of the year. To be sure, there are some days in August, for example, that may be too hot for comfort. And there are times during January and February that get downright cold. But pretty days occur the year around.

It was on one of those gorgeous days in December that Jack and I were having Saturday lunch on our patio and listening to the Metropolitan Opera radio broadcast. Except for overseas tours of duty in the Navy where the broadcasts were unavailable, Jack has made listening to these Texaco-sponsored events a ritual since his teenage years in the late 1940's.

Halfway into my turkey sandwich, I suddenly felt a terrible cramp on the right side of my neck. It was like being pinched by a giant clothespin. My mouth also felt as dry as dust. I decided to keep eating lunch, hoping and thinking the cramping would disappear as mysteriously as it had come.

A few minutes later, all of a sudden my neck started swelling. I must have looked like a gecko puffing up his neck during mating time. Jack looked at me in astonishment. "My Lord! What's happening to your neck?"

"I don't know, but it hurts like crazy," I replied, as puzzled as Jack was by the strange reaction. "Maybe something I've eaten caused my glands to secrete a lot."

"That doesn't make sense. You and I have been eating the same things," he responded with his usual logic.

A couple of hours later my neck was almost back to normal in size, but the soreness remained. I felt relatively sure my new malady wasn't anything too serious. However, Jack was not so sanguine. He seemed quite concerned and questioned me throughout the rest of the day as to how my neck was doing.

For the next couple of weeks, a slight swelling persisted. As chance would have it, we were eating lunch outdoors two Saturdays later when it happened all over again. First came the severe cramping, followed by my neck ballooning up.

Jack's reaction was immediate. "Mary, darlin', you've got to get yourself to the doctor right away and see what in the world is going on."

I agreed. Early Monday I called my new oncologist, Dr. Shildt. When I explained what had happened, he told me to come in that afternoon.

There are precious few advantages from having cancer, and everyone knows the obvious disadvantages. The lone advantage I've found is that once you've been diagnosed with the disease, no one procrastinates in trying to find the cause of a new pain or complaint.

By the time I reported to the Oncology Clinic, my neck was almost back to normal. Dr. Shildt, a man small in stature, but huge in kindness and in the typically attentive mold of most oncologists, examined me carefully. He detected a slight swelling on the right side of my neck and unhesitatingly referred me to the Eye, Nose, and Throat (ENT) Clinic.

It also has been my experience that once a person is diagnosed with cancer and goes to see a new doctor, that doctor is always very alert to any possible spreading and would rather err on the side of caution than overlook any new activity. And, of course, being referred by an oncologist just adds fuel to the speculation fire.

Later that week I reported to the ENT Clinic as scheduled. A slight, bespectacled man in his late thirties with thinning hair greeted me and introduced himself as Dr. Dickson.

After carefully examining me, the ENT doctor concluded that my right submandibular salivary gland was larger than normal. He instructed me to keep a close watch on the area. If the neck swelling occurred again, he wanted me to return to his clinic immediately so he could observe the ballooning phenomenon himself.

I left Dr. Dickson's office relatively assured that what had happened before was an anomaly and that I wouldn't have any more trouble.

It didn't take much time to dispel my optimism. About a week later, while eating again, I started to feel that unmistakable cramping in my neck. Within a few minutes, my neck blew up as big as a balloon. I facetiously thought that, given the right wind, I could have floated to the hospital like an air-filled dirigible.

After calling the ENT Clinic to get approval to come in, I

drove to the hospital. As I sat in what resembled a modified dentist's chair waiting for Dr. Dickson, I pondered my situation. "Oh, great God!" I thought. "I seem to take two steps forward and then go three steps backward. Surely this can't be the cancer again!"

Dr. Dickson looked surprised when he entered the room and saw me. "Oh, my! You really are swollen, Mrs. Walker!"

I nodded in agreement. "Not only am I swollen, but it hurts to eat and move my head."

"Let's take a look at it," Dr. Dickson urged as he began to examine my neck. After a very methodical examination, he sat down on a chair next to me. "You've got something blocking the tube leading from the right submandibular or salivary gland. I can't tell precisely whether it's a tumor or a stone. But whatever it is, we're going to have to find out."

"What does that entail?" I asked warily.

"That calls for surgery."

A feeling of deja vu swept over me as I heard the word "surgery" once again.

"We're going to have to remove your submandibular gland. The reason you're having so much swelling is because the saliva flow is blocked. When the gland is stimulated to secrete, the liquid has nowhere to go except to back up."

"Will losing that salivary gland interfere with my eating?" I wondered.

"It shouldn't. The other glands should pick up the slack, and you should do nicely with what you have left."

Dr. Dickson scheduled my surgery for a couple of weeks later and agreed to keep Dr. Shildt informed.

When I told Jack about the newest development, he was very apprehensive that any tumor in my gland might be malignant. A cautious person by nature, his love for me and fear of losing me to cancer was causing him to suspect every slight change in my physical condition as a return of the disease.

I awoke on the morning I was scheduled to check into the hospital with a stuffy nose and feeling bad. By the time I was undergoing my pre-operative physical, an intern discovered I was running a fever. Dr. Dickson immediately rescheduled the surgery for two weeks later. After diagnosing my illness as an upper respiratory infection, he decided to keep me in the hospital for a couple of days to treat me with antibiotics.

When I returned in two weeks, my cold and infection were gone. After completing my pre-operative tests again, Dr. Shildt came up to my ward and wished me good luck during the surgery. It was difficult to tell whether his relatively optimistic words truly reflected his thoughts or whether his oncologic background of comforting cancer patients stimulated his assuring words.

Early the next morning, in what by now was becoming far-too-commonplace a routine, I was pushed to the operating room on a gurney. As soon as the general anesthesia was injected, I was fast asleep.

I awoke a couple of hours later back in my bed on the ward, apparently spending no time in the recovery room. As usual, Jack was there to greet me from my slumber—like Siegfried greeted Brünnhilde after her long sleep.

About an hour after the anesthesia wore off, Dr. Dickson, accompanied by Dr. Shildt, approached Jack and me. Their faces were expressionless.

"Are you awake now, Mrs. Walker?" Dr. Dickson inquired.

"I'm a bit groggy, but I'm awake."

"The surgery went just fine," Dr. Dickson continued. "You had a tumor blocking your salivary duct. We removed the tumor along with your submandibular gland. You should recover nicely."

"Could you tell from the tissue if the tumor or gland was malignant?" Jack asked.

"Not really. We sent it all off to pathology. We should know something for sure in a couple of days."

After Dr. Dickson left the ward, Dr. Shildt reassured me that he would give me the pathological report as soon as it became available. In the meantime, he urged me not to worry.

"I won't, I'll leave that to Jack. He'll worry enough for both of us," I quipped.

I reached the conclusion long ago that it wasn't going to do me any good to worry anyway. Whatever is going to happen will happen. And if something bad happened again, it was my good fortune that medical professionals were trying to solve the problem and help me.

For the first time since my hysterectomy in 1973, I was able to roam around the ward unencumbered by wheelchairs, crutches, or slings. Consequently, I was able to socialize freely and meet the other patients on the ward. My only impediment was a fog-horn sounding voice which was a temporary side effect of my surgery. However, I fit in well with the rest of the ward, which reminded me of the characters in *Treasure Island*. Everyone had a bandage on her eye, neck, or ear. All one patient with a patch on her right eye needed was a parrot and a pegleg to look like Long John Silver.

The day after my surgery Dr. Dickson removed the bandage temporarily to check the incision. When I saw the scar, I exclaimed: "Gee, you did a terrific job. You cut right on a wrinkle. Now I won't have a turkey neck."

I could tell from Dr. Dickson's puzzled look he had no idea what I was talking about.

I explained I was referring to the droopy skin that hangs under a turkey's beak.

About mid-morning the next day Dr. Shildt appeared at my bedside. A big smile graced his face. "I've got good news, Mrs. Walker. The tumor was benign! You can go home as soon as Dr. Dickson releases you. Keep a close eye on everything, and make sure you keep me informed if you have any problems."

Four days later I was discharged, filled with the hope that I was once again moving forward and not sliding backward.

Chapter Thirty-One

"I hate to tell you this, Mrs. Walker, but you have pneumonia."

I couldn't believe Dr. Shildt's words as he examined my X-rays. It seemed impossible that once again I faced the prospect of returning to the hospital just three weeks after my gland surgery.

I couldn't mask my disappointment. "Please don't put me in the hospital again. I know I can take care of myself at home."

Dr. Shildt continued to ponder the X-rays and the radiologist's report as I begged him for a reprieve. Normally we would hospitalize you. But this time we'll do it your way. I'll put you on penicillin and trust you not to overdo."

"Thanks so much, Dr. Shildt. I'll do my best to follow your instructions."

"We need to get on top of this," Dr. Shildt stressed as he began writing my prescription. "I think this is a holdover from the upper respiratory infection you had last month before your surgery."

I spent the next two weeks close to home recuperating and tying up loose ends on my parents' upcoming fiftieth-wedding-anniversary celebration.

The Fat Lady Hasn't Sung

In addition to the anniversary party, Jack and I wanted the kids to see some of the Western national parks while we were in that part of the country.

In mid-June, armed with maps, brochures, games, and books, we drove to Mesa, Arizona, the first leg of our "excellent" adventure.

The anniversary party was a huge success. In addition to my parents' anniversary, Jack and I celebrated our 20th anniversary, and our niece, Melinda, was there on her honeymoon with a young man she had met and married in Texas.

After a few days in the Phoenix area, we headed out to Hoover Dam and Las Vegas, our first stop. We took in the floor show at Caesar's Palace, but David and Amy were too young to try their luck at the slot machines.

We gasped in awe at nature's artistry in Bryce Canyon and Zion National Parks in Utah. Our three days in Yellowstone National Park proved to be inadequate to grasp the enormous diversity of that national treasure.

As we began to head south toward the Grand Tetons, the siren call of shooting the rapids on the Snake River grew louder and louder for the kids and me. Although Jack was less than enthusiastic, he reluctantly agreed to accompany us.

David and Amy could barely restrain their zeal as we piled into the rubber raft which would take us into the churning fury of the Snake River. Since our weight had to be evenly distributed, our guide sat the kids and me aft, and he and Jack provided counterbalance up forward.

After outfitting us all with life jackets, the guide pushed us into the water with his long pole. The first 200 yards were relatively calm. But up ahead we could hear a roar and see the mist rising from the turbulence as the river inexorably rushed to lower elevations.

There was no turning back now as our raft followed the deepest channel of swirling water among huge boulders resting on the river's bottom. Our raft now was buffeting back and forth against the giant rocks like a cork floating in a rain-swollen stream.

Suddenly, the forward part of the raft dipped downward as we passed over a submerged stone, and a wall of icy water came over the bow, striking Jack directly in the face and chest. We had, in Navy parlance I long ago had learned from Jack, taken "green water over the bow." But this green water was different from the tropical oceans Jack had known from his Navy days. This water was 39 degrees and came from the recently-melted snow on the nearby Grand Teton mountain range.

Jack had an agonized expression on his face as he turned around to see if the kids and I were okay. From the smiles on our faces, he must have concluded that we were having a great time. He quickly turned back to face forward just in time to brace himself for the next onslaught of frigid water. The Snake River continued to pound Jack unrelentingly each time the raft hit a new wave.

Mercifully for Jack, our ride finally came to an end. The kids and I experienced a wonderfully exciting journey, while Jack was completely soaked, and was shivering like a cold pup. He changed clothes and hung his socks and underwear out the window to dry as we continued our journey to Cheyenne.

Instinctively, the kids and I never got up enough nerve to ask Jack to accompany us on another white-water adventure.

A couple of days later we were taking in the spectacular views of Rocky Mountain National Park in Colorado. We followed the Trail Ridge Road over passes of almost 12,000 feet above sea level. Even in July, there was still plenty of snow alongside the road for David and Amy to throw snow balls.

After three weeks of acute togetherness, all of us were overjoyed when we finally drove into our driveway, thus ending our Western excursion.

Because our grass had not been mowed since before we started our trip, it was almost a foot high when Jack broke out the lawn mower the next day. As the machine inched its way through the thick growth, miraculously Jack stopped just short of a rabbit's nest containing three new-born bunnies.

As soon as David and Amy saw the pink sucklings, the kids

began to beg their dad to keep them. They even promptly named them Thumper, Rufus, and Willamina. Without her long grass sanctuary, Jack realized there was no way mama cottontail would return again to take care of her babies. His choice was either to let them perish as orphans or attempt to save them with human intervention. Reluctantly, he acquiesced to the kids' urging.

While I busily obtained a special formula and food from the veterinarian, Jack began construction on a hutch. We all discovered that wild rabbits in captivity do not make good patients. We finally had to force feed the trio to keep them alive. Eventually, when the bunnies matured, Jack and I convinced the kids that we had to return them to nature. In a scene reminiscent of a Jack London novel, we set them free on a nearby ranch. For several years after that, every time I drove past that spot I wondered if Thumper, Rufus, and Willamina made it to raise their own families.

Shortly after returning from our Western trip, I reported to the Orthopedic Clinic for a routine follow-up appointment.

Dr. Stanton, the chief resident, peered over the top of his glasses as he interpreted my newest X-rays. "The acetabular component on your right hip has approximately two millimeters lucency at the cement bone interface."

"Would you mind translating that for me?" I wondered.

"That just means we are beginning to see some loosening of the plastic cup in the right side of the pelvis."

"That doesn't sound too good."

"It's a natural by-product of wear and tear. It's nothing to worry about right now. Just try not to fall," Dr. Stanton cautioned.

Six months later a new set of X-rays revealed the right hip was about the same. But this time there was a "moth-eaten appearance" on the left femur. Once again, I was cautioned to avoid falling.

To help ease the adjustment for David and Amy when we moved from Maryland to Texas, Jack kept alive their hope that after we got re-settled a horse could be in their future. Although David seemed only mildly interested, Amy's equine love affair continued unabated since her ride on Gunther Gebel-Williams' white stallion at the circus in 1974.

In order to test their true devotion to horses before making a purchase, Jack and I arranged for the kids to work part time on weekends at a local riding stable. After a couple of months of mucking stalls, heaving saddles, and grooming, David decided he would rather pursue other interests. But Amy's love of horses only increased.

About this same time, Jack and I began to yearn for the wide open spaces ourselves. Our half-acre lot in the city was beginning to feel far too confining, and, like Amy, I grew up loving horses as well. Therefore, we decided to start looking for some land in the country not too far away where we could keep a horse and ultimately build our dream home.

We looked at several properties during the spring of 1980. All were nice, but each was flawed in some way so as to dissuade us from buying. Finally, we found the property we had envisioned in our dreams about 16 miles further north from our home. A 500-acre ranch, owned by an elderly couple, was being divided into tracts of 20 or more acres. As one of the first few potential buyers to see the land, we had our choice of almost any part of the acreage. A gentle spring rain had fallen during the night before our visit, freshening the air and reviving the wild flowers. The sun was shining brightly as we walked across the newly-sprouted green grass of a meadow dotted with groves of ancient moss-covered live oak trees. Robins and cardinals sang as they playfully carried out their mating rituals.

In the center of all this beauty rose a small mesa or flat-topped hill. With great effort and Jack's help, we struggled to the top. Neither of us were prepared for the awesome panorama which unfolded before us. To the north we looked over the Guadalupe River valley far below in a sea of green treetops leading to a distant horizon and a pair of hills, referred to by the locals as Twin Sisters. In every other direction one could see the horizon without obstruction.

As we took in the gorgeous view, we reflected that the day

was Good Friday. Just as the hero of Wagner's *Parsifal* exclaimed at the beauty of the spring fields of the Spanish Pyrenees in the "Good Friday Spell," Jack and I marvelled at the Texas Hill Country. And, like Parsifal, we knew we had found our own Grail in the form of our future home site.

As soon as arrangements could be completed, we signed an earnest money contract for almost 40 acres of raw land with our hill approximately in the center. On the first of July we finally went to settlement.

During the next several months the four of us cleared brush, put in over a quarter mile of fencing, and had a well dug. The work was back breaking, but instinctively, Jack knew how to direct our efforts.

For Christmas that year we fulfilled Amy's dream by giving her Belle, a sorrel quarter horse. For the same amount of money, we purchased an iron horse—a dirt motorcycle—for David. As it turned out, both kids got what they wanted.

Keeping a horse turned out to be more of a problem than any of us had realized. We drove out to replenish Belle's hay and to feed her grain at least every other day during the week. We generally spent weekends at the ranch staying in a travel trailer which gave us a place to cook meals and to escape the heat or cold. During this time Jack designed and we helped him build a tack barn and corral.

By now Amy had become an excellent equestrian and wanted to compete in horse shows. Her rapport with Belle was complete, and it seemed all she had to do was think about a command and the horse executed it. The only problem was Belle was no show horse. She didn't have the conformation the judges prized. Jack teased Amy by saying Belle looked like a barrel with toothpicks for legs.

Amy's response was to continue to try to persuade her dad that she needed a more showable horse. Besides, as I pointed out to Jack, horses are very sociable animals, and Belle was showing definite signs of loneliness.

We provided Belle some temporary companionship when we

decided to breed her to a neighbor's handsome, chestnut-colored stallion named Model Cinnabar. If she wasn't a show horse, maybe her colt could be. Nature was not kind, and it took three attempts and an infusion of antibiotic drugs for Belle to get pregnant.

For Mother's Day Jack bought me a gorgeous two-year-old registered quarter horse mare named "Honey Bee." She had a long, slim body and a muscular chest. This horse was aptly named because her coat was the exact color of honey.

Since I physically wasn't able to ride, Amy quickly took over Honey, and, in short order, developed a relationship with her similar to the one she had with Belle. After several weeks of working with a trainer, Amy decided she was ready to show.

We soon discovered there's a lot more to showing a horse than just the animal and rider. In short succession we purchased a horse trailer, silver-trimmed tack gear, a new saddle, and special clothes for Amy. We also learned that show horses have to be groomed, trimmed, and clipped in specified ways right down to coloring their hooves—like polishing human shoes.

In addition, proper feeding routine is necessary to prevent foundering, multiple shots are required twice a year, and worming is necessary every three months. And, the most frustrating of all from Jack's standpoint, was loading and unloading the horse and pulling her trailer around the state.

Amy and Honey ended up winning several ribbons at various horse shows in both riding and halter events.

It was at this time more than ever before that I realized just how much Jack truly was a Renaissance man. More than anyone I have ever known, he has so many broad interests and is knowledgeable about such a great variety of subjects.

In November I reported to the OB-GYN Clinic for my yearly pap smear and examination. To say that it was difficult to conduct the exam with my radiated legs and artificial hips would be an understatement. Even though there was no way I could spread my legs to fit into the table's stirrups, Dr. Black, a resident, finally maneuvered me into a position to begin.

The Fat Lady Hasn't Sung

The exam seemed to take considerably longer than I had remembered them taking in the past. Dr. Black then excused himself and said he had to go out and check on something. A few minutes later he returned accompanied by an older doctor whom he introduced as Dr. Leman, head of the clinic.

Dr. Leman also examined me and asked about my cancer background. He thanked me for my patience and left the room with Dr. Black.

By the time I got dressed, Dr. Black returned. His face was somber as he spoke. "Mrs. Walker, there's a mass in the back of your pelvis. It wasn't there last year. But both Dr. Leman and I can easily feel it now."

I was shocked. I had been feeling so well, and I hadn't experienced any pain. Once again, as I reacted after hearing bad news several years earlier, his voice seemed to be coming from a long distance or from the bottom of a well.

I gazed at Dr. Black in silence as he concluded: "It looks like the histiocytic lymphoma may have returned."

Chapter Thirty-Two

Jack was heart-broken when he learned that my cancer might have returned.

"I was afraid this might happen," he reacted dejectedly. "I knew they shouldn't have taken you off chemotherapy so soon. How are they ever going to get it under control again?"

"Now, Jack, let's not hang crepe until we know exactly what we're dealing with," I reassured him. "The doctors have ordered several tests. We should know something definite after the holidays."

The first test in mid-December was a pelvic ultrasound. Just as the two OB-GYN doctors had discovered, the ultrasound pictures clearly revealed the presence of a mass in the right portion of my pelvis.

Dr. Shildt seemed genuinely puzzled by the test results. "I don't know how a mass of that size could appear so suddenly when we've been doing periodic scans all along. We'll have to do a biopsy to determine if it's benign or malignant."

With the Christmas holiday rush already upon us, January 7 was the first available time the biopsy could be scheduled.

Jack and I decided to go ahead with our planned holiday trip to Arizona in spite of the disconcerting news. While Jack drove, I played games with David and Amy and did some needlepoint.

We decided not to tell my parents about our latest concerns until there was more definitive information after the biopsy. Besides, it was bad enough for us to have to worry about it without causing my parents any additional, and perhaps needless, anxiety.

Our Christmas holidays in Arizona were a wonderful interlude from the reality which awaited us upon our return to Texas.

On January 6 I reported to the gynecology ward at the hospital. Because of the condition of my hips, Dr. Leman decided to perform the biopsy in the operating room with me under general anesthesia. The next day Dr. Leman obtained samples of the mass by vaginal incision.

As usual, Jack spent the time waiting for news of how I had fared by pacing around the waiting room. After I awoke from the anesthesia, he went back to work until later in the day when he picked me up to take me home.

Dr. Leman was noncommittal about his opinion of what the mass might be. He would only promise the pathological report in two or three days.

When I awoke the next morning, my body was stiff and sore. By bedtime, I felt like I had been on the receiving end of a wrecking ball. Every part of my body—muscles, bones, tendons, and ligaments—cried out in pain. Jack even had to help me lower my head onto my pillow because my neck and back muscles were so sore.

Both of us were frightened by the unknown. What mysterious malady could I be coming down with now? Jack was concerned that disturbing the mass during the biopsy could somehow have accelerated its spreading. I wasn't sure about the logic of his thesis. The only thing I knew with certainty was that I felt lousy.

By Monday I was feeling somewhat better when I called Dr. Leman to get the pathological report and to tell him about my strange soreness.

I waited apprehensively for the results when I heard his voice on the phone. "I just received the report, Mrs. Walker." The short silence which followed seemed like an eternity. "I'm happy to tell you the mass is necrotic tissue. There is no malignancy!"

After the elation of his news soaked in, I was puzzled by the report. "Doesn't necrotic mean dead?"

"Actually it does. It's a term we use to describe non-living or scar tissue."

Dr. Leman seemed as baffled by the findings as I was. Neither of us could understand how necrotic or scar tissue would suddenly form in the back of my pelvis. For now, we would just have to chalk it up as one of life's big mysteries.

Dr. Leman was not surprised by my discomfort, however. "In order to get a decent biopsy, we had to roll you up on your shoulders," he explained. "And you had to remain in that position for quite a while."

I must have used muscles I didn't know I had and put pressure on areas I don't normally lie on in order to feel the way I did. Happily, a week later, my discomfort was just an unpleasant memory.

As Amy neared her fifteenth birthday, her enthusiasm for horses began to wane. It was getting more difficult to get her to come out to the ranch on weekends, and she no longer wanted to devote a lot of time to caring for the horses. Although she wasn't yet allowed to date, we got the impression she had become more interested in the two-legged variety than the four-legged animal.

Amy's equine interests spiked temporarily again when Belle's colt was born early on a late spring morning. Like his sire, the new-born's coat was a beautiful chestnut color. His face bore a white, lightning-bolt shaped mark, and his right hind pastern was white. Combining his mother's and father's names, we called him "Bar Bell" or "Bar" for short. But the novelty of the baby horse soon wore off, and Amy returned to her earlier mood.

Because Honey was so well trained and we already had made such a large investment in the horses in time and money, Jack and I were totally frustrated by Amy's sudden recalcitrance.

The Fat Lady Hasn't Sung

What could I do, I wondered, to shame her into working with the horses again?

Suddenly it dawned on me that *I* could show Honey at the adult horse shows. Although I realized I couldn't compete in the riding events, I knew I could show her in the halter class.

When I broached the subject to Jack, he was incredulous. "Are you out of your mind, Mary? How are you going to get that horse into a trot?" he asked, referring to the requirement for a person showing at halter to run and lead the horse into a full trot.

"I can run well enough to do that," I assured him, even though my most recent orthopedic checkup revealed one hip was moth-eaten, and the other was loose.

"But what if you fall?" he insisted. "With your artificial joints, you'd end up as a torso with one arm."

Over time and with my persuasive powers, Jack's opposition slowly abated. He knew I was bull-headed, and I wouldn't give up.

We made all the arrangements to enter the south-Texas fall adult horse show in September. The day before the event we carefully groomed Honey, clipping her whiskers and trimming the fur in her ears as prescribed by protocol. Early on the morning of the show, we thoroughly shampooed and brushed her before loading her into the trailer. Upon arrival at the site, Jack unloaded her and brushed her again. He then painted her hooves and put on her silver-trimmed halter. Her honey-colored coat glistened in the morning sunshine.

Jack pinned my entry number on the back of my sky-blue Western-style shirt which contrasted with my tan cowboy boots and matching Western trousers. Faded blue jeans and a tee shirt wouldn't have worked here. Every entrant had to look the part as completely as his or her equine partner.

As I led Honey into the arena, I knew I was in potential trouble when I sank ankle deep into a combination of sand and sawdust covering the ground.

Honey and I joined approximately two dozen other horses and trainers or owners from all over the Southwest and lined up in a long row in front of the grandstands. As the judges proceeded down the line, each horse had to be "set up"—essentially the equivalent of standing at attention—as the judges approached.

When the judges were within a couple of horses from us, I gently tugged on Honey's halter to let her know I wanted her to set up. She immediately lined up all four hoofs and stood like a statue. Even when the judges encircled her, she never blinked an eye or turned her head.

Then came the moment of truth when the head judge told me to bring her to a trot. Ever since my hip surgery, I hadn't been able to raise my legs very high. Now I had the challenge of trying to run in sand while wearing boots.

"Come on Honey," I whispered softly to her as I tried to move my legs fast enough to have her go from a walk to a trot. Almost as if she understood my physical limitations, she broke into a fancy, short-stepped trot as I struggled to keep from falling flat on my face. As I ran through the sand I thought I looked like the character Festus in the television series "Gunsmoke." At least I felt like one leg was in a bucket.

At the peak of our run, I must have hit a low spot in the ground cover, and I could feel the momentum of my upper body going faster than my legs. In that instant, terrible thoughts raced through my head. I'm going to fall just as Jack had warned me! Will the prosthetic devices break away from my bones? How embarrassing to fall in front of all these spectators!

In the next nanosecond I remembered my thousand-pound partner trotting at my side. I pulled downward on Honey's lead as hard as I could knowing that if she obeyed my signal and lowered her head, I would end up on the ground. Instead, almost as if she knew my dilemma, Honey jerked her head upward with her muscular neck, pulling up the lead and supporting my upper body long enough for my legs to catch up and avoid a fall.

When all the horses had been inspected, we all lined up again in a long brown row of horse flesh to await the judges' verdict. After awarding the first five places, the judges stopped in front of Honey and me and presented us with the sixth-place ribbon. I was shocked! My goal was only to participate. I had absolutely no aspirations about winning a ribbon. After all, I was competing against horse breeders and trainers who made their living from horses.

I have wondered to this day if the judges truly found Honey in the top quarter of the show based on merit, if they felt sorry for me trying to show a horse in my condition, or if they awarded her for demonstrating the "horse sense" to keep me from falling.

In addition to regular check-ups by the oncologist (including bone scans) and by the orthopedists for loosening of my hip prostheses, I was now being followed regularly in gynecology for the mysterious pelvic mass.

By now, Dr. Leman had retired from the Army and had entered civilian practice in San Antonio. His replacement, Dr. Capon, ordered pelvic ultrasound studies in July and December of 1982. Both studies revealed the continued presence of the mass, but fortunately, it was not growing.

By March of 1983, I had lived with my artificial hips for almost eight years. After that length of time, even "normal" hip replacements start to show signs of wear. Consequently, I was hospitalized for eight days for a work up to check on suspected loosening of the left hip prosthesis.

It was during this time that I met Dr. Allan Bucknell, the new chief of the major joint clinic. He was a handsome, intense man with dark, piercing eyes. Dr. Bucknell seemed to take a great deal of interest in my case. Eventually, he felt, I would need reconstructive surgery on both hips. I was discharged with the recommendation to be careful and to use either a cane or crutches plus heel pads to diminish stress across my left and right hips.

During that same time I started having some strange episodes with my heart. I noticed periods of palpitations coupled with racing and skipping of beats. By now Dr. Shildt was returning to civilian life, and he was in the process of turning me over to Dr. McCracken, head of oncology, when my heart started acting up.

On my first visit to see him as a patient, Dr. McCracken was in a jovial mood. "I am very fortunate," he beamed. "I get to see all the 'wellies.'" That was his term for patients who had survived at least five years after ending chemotherapy and who were still in remission. When I told him about my heart, he immediately gave me a consultation slip to cardiology.

At the cardiology clinic, the staff prepared me for a MUGA scan—a nuclear dying of the heart muscle to see how efficiently it functions. It's a strange sensation to look up on a television-like screen and see one's heart beating almost as if it were independent of the rest of the body.

Dr. McCracken didn't seem surprised by the results of the scan and the cardiologists' report. "We are probably seeing some of the first signs of early toxicity of Adriamycin," he announced unemotionally.

As he talked, I recalled Dr. Deas' earlier comments about the cumulative effects of the drug which had saved my life but whose after-effects seemed destined to continue to influence how I would live.

Spring was especially beautiful that year. The median strip on the highway to our ranch was a river of wild flowers, especially bluebonnets. Bar, almost a year old now, was as tame as a pup and looked forward to the carrots or apples he got as a treat every time we visited.

Jack mowed our lawn once a week during the growing season, and I helped by sweeping the grass from the sidewalks and driveway. One early evening in July, Jack was using his line trimmer, and I was working about 50 feet away. As I was sweeping, I inadvertently stepped off the sidewalk at an angle into the grass about three inches lower down. Instantaneously, I knew I was going to fall. I caught some of my weight with my arms, but my knees hit the sidewalk full force. Jack heard the "splat" of the bone hitting concrete from his location in the back of the yard and came running to help.

It was almost dark as Jack helped me into the house. My hips and shoulder seemed to be intact, and I reassured him that I would be all right and didn't need to go to the hospital. But when I awoke in the middle of the night, my knee had swollen to nearly double its normal size. It was impossible to bend it.

Early the next morning Jack drove me to the hospital. Fortunately, Dr. Bucknell already was there when we arrived. He took one look at my distended knee and ordered X-rays.

When we returned with the films, Dr. Bucknell ushered us both into an examining room. As he arranged the X-rays on the viewer, his benign facial expression turned to a frown. "You've fractured your patella," he began. My suffering through comparative anatomy at Mankato State hadn't been in vain as I realized he was referring to my knee cap. "I don't want to operate unless it's absolutely necessary. Do you think you can tolerate a cast?"

"I think so," I replied optimistically.

Dr. Bucknell personally supervised the casting which involved a full leg cast—from groin to heel. Obviously, with the cast I couldn't bend my leg at all, and getting into the car to go home was the first of many challenges with my new companion.

A couple of days later, after the swelling had eased, I went back to see Dr. Bucknell because the cast was sliding up and down my leg as I walked.

After examining the bright red skin on my heel, Dr. Bucknell expressed concern. "You're about to get a blister which could get infected," he explained. "And an infection in either of your legs could spread to your hip prosthesis. Then we *would* be in trouble."

With the doctor's supervision, the corpsmen in the cast room fabricated a device like a garter belt which encircled my waist and snapped onto the cast to hold it in the correct position and keep it from sliding up and down.

I struggled with the hard cast for eight weeks until a soft cast (with velcro fasteners which allowed removing for showers) replaced it for three more weeks. When the casts were finally removed, I had to undergo several weeks of physical therapy to rehabilitate my leg. By late fall, I was able to function normally once again.

Ever since my sister's move from Arizona to Texas, Jean and I had become increasingly concerned about our parents' welfare.

Dad's health continued to deteriorate, and by now Mom and Dad were approaching their mid-seventies. Finally, after much encouragement, they decided to move to Texas. They chose to live in Georgetown, near Jean, because they figured Jack had enough worries with me plus his responsibilities to his own mother who was now almost ninety.

During the fall Jean and I drove to Mesa to help Mom and Dad pack and get organized for their move. After the movers loaded their household effects into a van, we caravaned back to Texas with Dad riding with me and Jean and my mother driving our folks' car.

My joy at having all my family in Texas was short-lived. After the new year began, Dad's health got much worse. Following several tests, he was diagnosed as having esophageal cancer. All of us were stunned. We knew he had been failing, but we didn't realize how much. Because of his breathing problems, caused by severe asthma and emphysema, he was a poor surgical risk. Therefore, the only cancer treatment deemed available to him was radiation therapy.

For the next six weeks, my sister and I alternated driving Dad for daily radiation treatments at the Scott and White Hospital in Temple. But even with this effort, he seemed to be getting worse before our eyes.

In the meantime, I was due for another MUGA scan in March. The cardiologist noted a diminished left ventricular function from the previous scan. He speculated that it was caused by progressive cardiotoxicity from Adriamycin.

During this time I went to Georgetown as often as possible to see Dad and to give my mother moral support. It was a terrible strain on all of us—but particularly on Mom—to see my father waste away before our eyes. All of his food had to be blended because swallowing was becoming increasingly difficult.

Dad and I often discussed both his and my cancer. Ever since my initial diagnosis ten years earlier, Dad always told me he wished it could have been him instead of me. Now I could truthfully reciprocate his feelings. I told him I wished I could have had his kind. Unlike Dad, in view of my track record, I would likely have survived the surgery which might provide the cure that he was finding so elusive.

During all these difficult times, my father never showed any signs of rancor or bitterness. He blamed no one but himself for all his years of smoking.

In spite of Dad's problems, my own medical history continued to be written.

A routine follow-up sonogram test revealed the mass in my pelvis had increased about 40 percent in size and had changed shape since the last examination. That immediately sent up a caution flag to Dr. Capon who ordered another biopsy for early June.

I tried to put the best face possible on this new development around Jack, who, predictably, was quite disconsolate. But even I, in moments of self-doubt, began to wonder if this dreaded disease which was taking such a devastating toll from my father was about to go another round with me as well.

Chapter Thirty-Three

The feeling of emptiness I experienced as I hung up the telephone was the most profound of my life.

Jean had just called to tell me Dad passed away ten minutes earlier.

My sense of vacuity stemmed not only from losing my father but also from not having been able to be with him during his final hours.

The last month of my father's life was extremely difficult for all of us. He fell and broke his shoulder, which complicated caring for him. Because of lack of oxygen to his brain, he suffered several seizures and became quite disoriented on occasions. And he was in and out of the hospital several times.

I continued going to Georgetown as often as my own medical schedule and the needs of my husband and children permitted.

On June 4 I checked into BAMC for a biopsy of the pelvic mass. The next day I was discharged to await the biopsy results. On the following day came Jean's telephone call.

I think about Dad often, and I know I always will. And all of my thoughts are pleasant. Like most kids, I grew up with a hero.

The Fat Lady Hasn't Sung

But my hero wasn't a sports or movie star. My hero was my dad. From earliest childhood I always wanted to emulate Dad's traits of patience, kindness, understanding, and open-mindedness. Whether or not I ever achieved that goal remains to be seen. But there will never be any doubt in my mind that David Crawford was one of the most wonderful and thoughtful fathers anyone ever had.

My feeling of emptiness from Dad's death still shrouded me like a cloak when the phone rang again.

I recognized Dr. Capon's voice immediately. "We have the results of your biopsy," he began.

Although I had prepared myself psychologically for bad news, coming so quickly after hearing about Dad, I prayed for a favorable report as I awaited the rest of his words.

"Your pelvic mass is fibrosis only. There is no malignancy!"

Dr. Capon's report came as a much-needed balm at a very difficult time for me. Nothing could ever make up for losing Dad. But at least, to our knowledge, cancer was not stalking me again at this time.

The etiology of that mysterious pelvic mass would have to be discovered sometime in the future.

Our son, David, graduated from high school in 1984 and started his life's great adventure.

Now with only Amy at home, Jack and I started thinking more seriously about building our dream home on our ranch. But our plans didn't go beyond the imagination stage, since Amy still had another year of high school, and we didn't want to disrupt her by moving before her graduation.

That summer I noticed that a couple of spots on my back seemed to itch most of the time. After examining them, Jack thought they might be dry spots from daily swimming and chlorine exposure. But lotions and moisturizers didn't seem to help.

The dermatologist agreed the spots were troublesome and decided to perform a biopsy.

When I called to find out the results of the pathological report, the doctor was direct. "You have basal cell skin cancer,

Mrs. Walker."

Once one has been diagnosed with having cancer, the "C" word does not carry the same frightening connotations as it does upon initial diagnosis. But cancer is cancer, and I was both dismayed and surprised.

I was never much of a sun worshiper, and skin cancer is almost always the result of prior excessive sun exposure. The only real sunburns I can remember came when I was a teenager in Iowa detasseling corn for two summers wearing only shorts and a halter top. That early damage must be manifesting itself now as skin cancer 30 years later.

After a short pause in which I regained my composure, the doctor continued. "You need to come in for surgery as soon as we can schedule it."

Surgery for basal cell skin cancer consists of numbing the skin around the site with novocaine, scraping down the skin in the area several layers, and otherwise cutting out the cancerous tissue and the surrounding skin. All of this is done as an outpatient in a doctor's office.

After my surgery, Jack dressed the wounds daily with hydrogen peroxide and Bacitracin ointment. After about three weeks, the spots had healed nicely from the inside out. A couple of months later, only two small scars served as reminders of this round in my battle with cancer.

During the latter part of 1984, Jack and I decided now was the time to complete the plans for building on our ranch property. We had thought about it in the past, but Dad's death gave us the impetus we needed to start the wheels in motion. He had worked unbelievably hard for 50 years. But when retirement came, he never really had a chance to enjoy his new life because his poor health didn't permit it. Although we were still relatively young, my health was uncertain, and Jack and I were determined to accomplish what we had dreamed of while we were able to enjoy it together.

Shortly after the new year began, we started working with a local designer and builder to complete the blueprints for our new home. Although it's not too popular in the Southwest, we decided on a modified Greek revival style of architecture to be built all on one level. During these design sessions, I didn't think we could afford certain features which were suggested. But Jack insisted that this was the last house we would ever build, and if we wanted something, we should put it into the plans. That "something" even included an indoor pool so I could exercise year-round.

When our design was complete, we found out we could afford the extras. We signed a contract with a builder, and ground was broken on our dream home.

Simultaneously, we put our home in San Antonio up for sale in March with the knowledge that Amy would graduate in May, and she wouldn't have to be uprooted from school during her senior year.

Amy's graduation came on schedule. We both felt a sense of relief that we had gotten both our children through high school at least, and they were on their way to independence.

The real estate market in Texas was just starting to feel the effects of recession, and although several people looked at our home during spring and early summer, no one seemed interested enough to talk price or submit a contract.

Our Realtor convinced us that in order to sell we needed to update our home with new carpeting and brighter wallpaper in the entrance hall and dining room.

Neither of us realized what an undertaking recarpeting a home is. Several days before the installation team arrived, Jack and I emptied all our closets since the carpet there too had to be replaced.

On Saturday night before the carpet layers were scheduled to arrive on Monday, I got up in the middle of the night to go to the bathroom. While I was returning to bed, I must have stepped wrong or caught my foot on the carpet because I felt a sudden, terrible pain in my left thigh. I struggled to get back in bed without waking Jack by hopping on my right leg and hanging onto furniture. After a couple of hours of enduring severe pain, I finally drifted back to sleep.

The next morning I couldn't put any weight on my leg at all. Jack was concerned. "Why don't we go straight to the hospital and check out what's wrong?"

But I thought I could tough it out one more time. "Just get me my crutches, please; I'll be all right," I reassured him. "Besides, we've got to go to the Walker reunion today. And I'll be having my hip revised in August anyway."

For the past year and a half Dr. Bucknell had carried my X-rays to specialists all over the world to help him decide what to do about my failing hip joints. Some of those experts even visited San Antonio to examine me and consult on my case. After all this research, Dr. Bucknell decided to proceed first with reconstruction of the left femur and hip using bone grafts and a long-stemmed prosthesis.

I felt confident I could stay on crutches for the next seven weeks or so until I checked into the hospital for my hip reconstruction. I also figured the carpet installation would be complete and perhaps even the house might be sold by then. And I knew Jack needed my assistance to help accomplish those things.

My most immediate problem was dressing for the reunion. My left foot was so swollen I couldn't get my shoe on. I also couldn't apply any pressure to push my foot into the shoe due to excruciating pain which radiated up my leg.

"We don't need to go," Jack offered. "I'll call and let them know why we can't come."

"I'd like to try to go, Jack. Would you help me put on this shoe?"

"Forget about shoes, Mary, darlin'. Why don't you just wear bedroom slippers?"

"I haven't even met some of your relatives, Jack. They're going to think I'm some kind of hippy wearing slippers."

I persisted, and finally after much trying, struggling, and tears, we jammed my foot into my shoe. Jack borrowed a wheelchair, and we went to the reunion. In spite of my discomfort, we had a wonderful day. I met some of Jack's relatives for the first time and finally was able to match names and faces.

Early Monday morning a four-man carpet installation crew arrived ready to start their project. They swarmed over our house like bees, ripping up the old carpet from all the edges and corners and rolling the floor covering into large log-like cylinders in the middle of every room.

With me on crutches, just getting from one room to another proved to be an obstacle course.

When lunch time neared, I offered to make each man a sandwich since there were no restaurants nearby. They eagerly accepted my invitation.

After making their sandwiches, I placed them on paper plates and stacked them four high as I attempted to crutch and carry the food to the workmen while maneuvering through the rolls of carpet. Between the kitchen and the bedrooms where the men were working lay an enormous roll of carpet, stretching from wall to wall. Because there was no way I could raise my legs up high enough to hurdle the roll, I had no choice but to get on top of the roll with my crutches and then try to lower myself to the other side. Once I was on top of the roll, I felt like a lumberjack on a log rolling in the water of the Pacific Northwest because the roll started to turn. I suddenly had visions of falling and lying flat on my back on the floor with bologna sandwiches all over my chest.

Fortunately, one of the men saw my dilemma and came to my rescue, catching me before I had a chance to fall off the roll.

After two days of carpet laying, the workmen finally finished their job, and we were able to get the house back in some sort of show condition.

Jack and I decided to do the wallpapering ourselves since we had done it successfully before. By the time we selected the paper and got our supplies together, it was almost time to check into the hospital for my upcoming reconstructive surgery. Of course, traveling to and from our ranch each day to check on the progress of our new home took a lot of our time as well.

We had just started replacing the wallpaper in the dining room when I checked into BAMC on August 1.

Dr. Bucknell requested that I come in early to complete all my pre-operation tests. Once finished, I was told I could go home for the weekend on pass until my surgery early the next week.

In addition to chest and hip X-rays, blood work, and other routine tests, Dr. Bucknell wanted me to have a gynecological exam and have my teeth checked to make sure I didn't have any cavities or anything else which could cause an infection.

The oral surgeon who checked my teeth and gums was impressed with my dental hygiene. He praised me for the condition of my teeth saying I had the gums of a person 25 years old.

The gynecological examination was a bit more challenging. Due to the pain in my leg, I couldn't get into the stirrups. The physician tried to conduct his exam under those conditions but speculated that he couldn't do a very thorough check because I couldn't spread my legs and I was in such pain.

Finally, in a stroke of mutual creativity, we decided I would put my legs up on his shoulders, and he would do the exam that way.

Fortunately, no other medical personnel other than the attending female corpsman entered the room during that time or they might have gotten the wrong idea.

As he took a Pap smear, he chuckled and said: "I can hardly wait to get home tonight to tell my wife about this. I normally always tell her my day was routine."

We both laughed at the bizarre situation we found ourselves in.

As he gave me the rest of the exam, he said, "Mrs. Walker, you have an extremely tight anal sphincter muscle. It's like an 18-year-old boy's."

I couldn't resist the irony of the situation. "That's great, doctor," I began. "I've got 25-year-old gums and an 18-year-old sphincter! I'm great at both ends. But I'm sure falling apart in the middle."

With all my tests complete, but not evaluated, Dr. Bucknell agreed to let me go home Friday afternoon with orders to return Sunday night with surgery scheduled for Tuesday.

I was delighted with the chance to come home and spend some time with Jack before the long ordeal ahead of me. Although Jack wasn't too keen about me helping, I also figured we could finish up the wallpapering in the dining room before I had to return to the hospital.

We were just sitting down to a magnificent fillet mignon dinner which Jack had prepared in honor of my return home when the phone rang.

Wanda White, one of the civilian nurses on the orthopedic ward, was on the line.

"Mrs. Walker, you've got to come back to the hospital right now," she urged with a hint of desperation in her voice.

"But Wanda," I said incredulously, "Dr. Bucknell told me I could come home. I've checked out officially. I'm just sitting down to dinner."

"You've got to come back *now*," Wanda persisted.

"What on earth is wrong? Why come back now?"

"I can't tell you. But you must come back now."

"I've done everything Dr. Bucknell asked me to do. I can't understand it. Would you have someone call me to explain it?" I asked.

"I've got someone right here beside me who would like to talk to you," Wanda responded.

A male voice which I didn't recognize spoke next. "Mrs. Walker, this is Dr. Olson." When I heard his name I remembered him as a new intern who was on rotation to orthopedics. "I'm part of Dr. Bucknell's team. You've got to come back. You've got a broken femur in your left leg!"

"It couldn't be broken, Dr. Olson. It doesn't hurt that bad."

"Please, Mrs. Walker. Please come back tonight," he pleaded. "If Dr. Bucknell and his staff find out I let you go home without checking those X-rays, my head will roll. I'll have to go back to med school!"

"May I at least finish dinner?"

"Okay," he agreed reluctantly. "But be back here before 10 p.m. Please promise me you will."

I promised him I would.

Jack and I were both disappointed as we resumed our now cold dinner.

When we finished eating, I looked at the clock. "We've got a couple of hours, Jack. Let's do what wall papering we can."

CHAPTER THIRTY-FOUR

Early the next morning I got out of my hospital bed and crutched into the community bathroom.

I was just starting to brush my teeth when I heard a frantic voice at the nurses' station nearby.

"Where's Mrs. Walker? She's not in her bed! Where is she?"

"I don't know," the nurse on duty responded. "She checked back in last night. She's got to be around here someplace."

I stopped brushing my teeth and poked my head out the door. "I'm right here," I shouted toward the vociferous pair at the counter. "I'll be right out."

When I finished up in the bathroom and started out, the slightly-built man who had been looking for me approached. He was clad in the white coat of a physician. "Mrs. Walker, I'm Dr. Olson. I want to thank you so much for coming back last night."

"You're welcome, Dr. Olson," I replied, somewhat taken aback by such unusual courtesy from a doctor. "But I want you to prove to me that my leg is broken. I can't believe I've been stumping around on crutches for two months with a broken femur."

Dr. Olson escorted me to the X-ray viewing room and arranged my pictures along the lighted panel. As I gazed at the shadowy images, even to my untrained eye it was obvious the bone was broken. Not only was the femur fractured, but the bones were offset.

Dr. Olson explained that since the break was near the middle of the femur instead of up by the head where the prosthetic device was, my scheduled surgery might have to be postponed. He would, of course, defer to Dr. Bucknell's judgment.

When Dr. Bucknell came in for his weekend rounds, I never let on that I had experienced a few hours of freedom away from the hospital Friday night. I let him believe that his staff had discovered the fracture just in time to prevent me from leaving his orthopedic ward with a broken leg.

Dr. Bucknell didn't seem overly concerned about the discovery. He said the fracture wouldn't make any difference because he had to shore up the entire length of the femur anyway. He previously had discussed the mechanics of the surgery with Jack and me. His plan was to get sufficient bone from the bone bank (since so many of the areas from which I might normally be able to donate my own bone had been radiated) to graft to and to strengthen my femur much like staves in a barrel. A new, long-stemmed prosthesis would be inserted to provide stability. Hopefully, the donor bone would unite with and take to my existing bone once the surgeons had removed my present device.

Dr. Bucknell assured me that I was still on target, that all my tests came back normal, and that I would be the first patient on the operating schedule for Tuesday.

I felt good as I took my shower Monday night. I scrubbed my left leg and side thoroughly with betadine soap and then left the reddish-brown suds on my skin to dry as instructed. My attitude was upbeat. I was confident that Dr. Bucknell's plan—the culmination of months of planning with input from the world's best orthopedic surgeons—was going to work. I was positive that when our new house was finished I'd be walking around without crutches. Then, when my left leg was stable and could support my weight, I would have my other leg revised. Maybe, then, I'd be like a "real" person again.

About 5:30 the next morning I was riding a gurney—by now an increasingly familiar mode of transportation—to the operating room. Naked as the day I was born under green surgical sheets, that familiar blast of cold air chilled me as the OR doors opened to embrace me once again.

The OR nurse fitted my head with a designer bonnet as the anesthesiologist discussed his plan. Over near the operating table I saw Dr. Bucknell, completely attired in his surgical garb, along with at least a half dozen other orthopedic surgeons and residents.

"Okay, Mary, we'll see you after it's all over." Dr. Bucknell said. "You'll be in intensive care at least overnight. Perhaps even a bit longer since this exact procedure has never been done before."

"God bless you, Dr. Bucknell," I said as the anesthesiologist began his routine. "I have every confidence. . ."

When I awoke in intensive care several hours later, I looked around to get my bearings. My leg hurt some, but I wasn't in great pain. As soon as I was alert enough to recognize people, Dr. Bucknell came over to my bed.

"How do you feel, Mary?"

"Pretty good. How did it go?"

"The surgery went well. Mechanically, we did everything just as we planned it. However, your bone was not what we anticipated."

"Why? What was wrong with it?"

"Mary, your bone is like a cadaver's bone. It doesn't even have the look of live bone. It has no color, probably no minerals."

"Is that from all the radiation?"

"I'm afraid so. I only hope it has enough vigor left to unite with the bone graft," Dr. Bucknell concluded, as the weariness of five and a half hours of surgery was now showing in his eyes.

Before he departed, Dr. Bucknell allowed Jack to come into intensive care to visit me for a few minutes. Despite his cheerful exterior, Jack looked as tired as Dr. Bucknell after all the waiting and uncertainty.

The intensive care staff kept me comfortable during my stay there, and, 24 hours later, I was back on the orthopedic ward.

Ever since coming out of the operating room, my leg was heavily bandaged, in a sling, and in traction. The master plan was for me to remain on my back, essentially motionless, for six to eight weeks to allow the bone graft to take. I must have looked like one of those ski accident victims in those funny cartoons.

My left thigh looked huge from all that extra bone along with some swelling. I joked with the other women on the ward that once I recovered from this surgery, I'd be able to kick field goals in the NFL since I had such a big leg.

It was good to be back on the ward. Jack, of course, visited me every day in addition to doing his job, supervising the construction of our new house, trying to sell our current home, and keeping track of our kids. David and Amy also visited often. The Navy wives of San Antonio, relatives, and our neighbors also were quite attentive.

Several days after the surgery, Dr. Bucknell came by to tell me he was leaving town for a medical convention in Europe and that he would be gone between ten days and two weeks. He said he was leaving the chief resident in charge.

His tone was firm as he gave me instructions. "Mary, if anything happens or if something turns up while I'm gone, don't let *anybody* take *anything* out of that leg!"

"What do you mean?" I questioned, unable to grasp his underlying concern.

"I don't want any of the grafted bone removed. Just say 'no.' *Nothing* is to be taken out of the leg."

Naturally, I didn't see that there would be any reason for that to happen. "No problem, Dr. Bucknell," I assured him. "I'll follow your instructions. Have a great time in Europe!"

Several days later, while making rounds, the surgical team seemed to take an uncommon interest in my incision. By now the large pressure bandage had been removed, but drainage tubes were still in place. The doctors took turns looking at my wound and even smelling the light bandage covering the area.

"What's going on," I asked.

"We don't know," the chief resident replied. "But something is seeping from your incision. We'll have to take a culture of this," he added as he sniffed the bandage again.

I began to feel progressively worse. I seemed to be tired all the time, and it was difficult to stay awake. My appetite fell off. Each time the nursing staff took my vitals, I would have a spiked temperature.

Every morning during rounds the doctors appeared to be more and more concerned about the seepage from my incision. By now, the liquid had taken on an unpleasant odor.

The lab report of the culture contained the dreaded news: I had developed an infection. The medical staff started me on oral antibiotics immediately, and I was confident that through the miracle of modern drugs I would soon be all right again.

By now Jack had finished wallpapering in what spare time he had. But very few potential buyers were looking, and we were getting a little concerned about selling our home. Since we needed the money from the sale of our present house to help pay for the cost of the new one, Jack started looking into the feasibility of a bridge loan.

As the days passed, I continued to feel increasingly worse. Finally, about two weeks after my surgery, the chief resident came by one evening. "We need to take you to the OR tomorrow morning," he announced.

"Oh, no! Dr. Hudson," I exclaimed. "Dr. Bucknell said nobody should take anything out of that leg."

"We're not taking anything out. But we need to go in and debride the wound."

"Debride?"

"Yes, we need to open up your leg and wash it out with an antibiotic solution to help get on top of this infection."

"Well, okay, I guess. As long as you don't take anything out."

"I just talked to Dr. Bucknell in Europe, and he concurs," Dr.

Hudson revealed. "Our plan is to debride the wound with you under general anesthesia and then bring you right back here to the ward."

Because of the danger of spreading my infection, I had to be the last person on the operating room schedule the next day. Consequently, I wasn't allowed to eat anything after midnight. Finally, about 4:30 p.m., I was wheeled off to the OR and put to sleep. The surgeons laid open the fourteen-inch incision all the way down to the bone. They washed out the bone and grafts and all the surrounding tissue with antibiotics, packed the wound with sterile bandages, wrapped my leg up tight, and brought me back to the ward.

The ward staff saved my dinner tray for me. Although I hadn't eaten in 24 hours, I had no appetite, and I felt somewhat nauseated from the anesthesia. Despite Jack's urgings, I was only able to pick at my food.

The next day the chief resident announced I might have to go back to the operating room the next day.

"I was just in there yesterday," I reminded him.

Dr. Hudson nodded. "I know. But we may have to do this every other day. It looks like the infection has gotten to the grafted bone."

Once again, after all the other patients had cleared the OR for the day, I was back for another debridement session under general anesthesia. Again, I went without food for about 24 hours, and, again, I wasn't hungry when I finally could eat.

During about my fourth debridement session, I heard a familiar voice greeting me. "I'm sorry this happened, Mary," Dr. Bucknell began. "But we're going to get on top of it."

By now I had become a very familiar character to the OR staff. I was there so often that they all knew my first name. Every other afternoon they could count on Mary Walker coming in one more time to get washed out.

As soon as Dr. Bucknell returned he ordered more cultures of the infection. Past attempts to grow a culture were either negative or non-specific.

Finally, Dr. Bucknell received the definitive laboratory report he had awaited. He was glad to finally know what germ he was dealing with. But he was clearly unhappy about the kind.

"Mary, your infection is called *Pseudomonas*," Dr. Bucknell explained.

"That sounds terrible. How could I have caught that?"

"It's a hospital-incurred infection. While we had your leg open for over five hours, the bacteria somehow invaded your system and has taken hold of you."

"How serious is it?" I wanted to know.

"It's pretty serious. It can even be life-threatening. We're going to have to do some major things to get this under control."

The first thing was to order stronger oral antibiotics. The second was to move me to the quarantine area—a spot at the far end of the ward behind a storage area and out of visual contact with the other people on the floor. I was the lone sick person, and the area was strictly off-limits for all the other patients since their surgical wounds might be vulnerable to the *Pseudomonas* bacteria. Of course, I could still have visitors, and the staff continued to care for my needs.

A new chief resident, Dr. Christianson, took over those duties during this time. He demonstrated a deep interest in my case and regularly reported my status to Dr. Bucknell when the latter was unavailable.

Every 48 hours I returned to the operating room for another debridement session under general anesthesia. Under those conditions, what little appetite I had completely disappeared. My weight continued to drop, and I was totally debilitated.

My high hopes for being able to walk again were being eclipsed by my struggle to get on top of the infection and survive.

For only the second time since my bout with cancer started in 1974, I was sinking into a depression.

When Jack made his daily visit that night, he looked almost as exhausted as I felt. Each day he had to have our home in show condition, check on the builders of our new house, prepare for his new classes which had just started, ride herd on our two children, and visit me. I felt like events beyond our control were crushing us.

Shortly after his arrival, I burst into uncharacteristic tears. "I'm never going to get on top of this," I sobbed.

Jack comforted me with his strong embrace. "Of course you will, Mary darlin'. Of course you will!"

But even with Jack's love and reassurance, my depression was too deep-seated to reverse.

"No matter what I try, it doesn't seem to help. The antibiotics haven't done anything. All that debriding hasn't made a difference."

As I wept, Jack quietly reassured me of his love.

"Here I've beaten cancer. But it looks like this stupid infection is going to end up getting me after all."

CHAPTER THIRTY-FIVE

Jack decided to do something positive to help relieve my depression. As soon as possible after visiting me, he contacted my new oncologist, Dr. Brown. Jack explained my situation and asked him to visit me.

I was surprised the next morning when Dr. Brown showed up at my bedside. He was a kind, gentle man whose head reflected the advanced stage of male-pattern baldness.

As I might have expected from an oncologist, he was very understanding and full of empathy. "Mrs. Walker, you've beaten the biggest disease of all. This infection is something we can treat. And we *will* treat it."

"But it's been going on so long," I reminded him.

"It just takes a while to get the right medicine. It's sort of like chemotherapy. As you well know, we've got to get the right recipe. But you have to keep up your attitude and remain determined that you're going to beat this infection just as you conquered cancer."

Dr. Brown's words made me feel better. More importantly, I decided he was absolutely right. I wasn't going to let this infection lick me.

Although my psychological outlook improved, my infection had not.

By now I had gone to the operating room twelve times over the past four weeks. Each time, under general anesthesia, my bone and surrounding tissue were washed out.

Unfortunately, the infection wasn't getting any better.

Finally, Dr. Bucknell decided enough was enough. During rounds the next day he announced his decision. "We're not taking you to the OR and putting you under anesthesia anymore for debridement. It's too hard on your heart and everyone concerned. Do you think you could stand having us do the debridement here on the ward at your bedside?"

"I suppose so," I replied apprehensively.

The next day, the surgical team showed up at my bed with all their paraphernalia. They carefully unwrapped my leg, revealing an angry open wound which extended from my left buttock to almost my knee. Then they removed the surgical packing from inside, revealing most of my grafted femur bone. If I had been weak-stomached, the sight of such a gaping opening in one's own body might have caused me to faint or at least made me sick.

As they washed, cleaned, and scraped inside my leg, surprisingly it didn't hurt much. Only when they touched semi-live bone did I feel any real discomfort. But when they contacted the grafted bone, it felt like they were touching an inanimate object.

After about a half dozen bedside debridements, both Dr. Bucknell and Dr. Christianson became more pessimistic about getting the infection out of the bone.

That evening after rounds, Dr. Bucknell reached into my leg cavity and broke off a piece of the grafted bone. He held it up for me to see. The bone was dark and discolored. It looked like something Snoopy might have buried to chew on at a later time.

"The bone graft isn't going to work, is it?" I asked tentatively, not really wanting to hear his inevitable reply.

Dr. Bucknell stared at the lifeless bone for a long time before answering. His face had the look of an artist whose masterpiece had just been destroyed by a disaster. "No, Mary, I really don't think it will," he said reluctantly. "Our only alternative now is to go back to the OR and take it all out."

I thought about my investment of lying on my back in traction for six weeks with all the attendant discomfort as I pleaded a hopeless cause. "But what will I have to walk on if we do that?"

"We'll put in a rod or do something else," Dr. Bucknell assured me. "But let's get rid of the bone and get on top of this infection now. We can worry about what we put in there after we get it cleaned up."

For the thirteenth time since I checked into the hospital in August, I was on my way to the operating room again. Under general anesthesia, the surgical team removed all of the grafted bone and most of my now crumbling femur as well. Since the infection had gone into the surrounding tissue of my leg, the doctors could not close the wound. Instead, they filled the void with surgical packing and wrapped my leg with bandages. That way they could continue the debridement of the wound until the infection was over, and it could begin to heal from the inside out. They continued to keep my empty leg in traction to prevent shrinkage in anticipation of eventually inserting a metal rod.

The bedside debridement continued every other day for the next several weeks. Without bone in my thigh, this procedure soon became quite routine and was relatively painless.

With the infection still raging, my appetite was nonexistent. In spite of urgings from Jack, the doctors, and the hospital staff, I couldn't eat more than a few bites during mealtimes.

I continued to lose weight dramatically. From 105 pounds in August, I was down to about 85 pounds in late September. I commented to one of the nurses urging me to eat that I could be front and center in the *Danse Macabre* because I looked like such a skeleton.

Mother and Jean brought a cake and visited me on my birthday. Although they treated me as though nothing was wrong, I found out later they both cried all the way back to Georgetown because they thought I would die from the infection.

The pounds continued to slip away as the infection sapped my strength and dulled my appetite. I now weighed 75 pounds.

One day Dr. Christianson showed up with three new faces with him. He introduced them as Dr. Stewart, a hematologist he had known since med school, and Doctors Short and Mobley from the infectious disease department.

The four doctors discussed my case with me in depth, including my weight loss, my lack of response to oral antibiotics, and my deteriorating veins which made it almost impossible to draw blood or insert an i.v.

They all agreed, without saying as much in my presence, that something dramatic had to be done quickly to save my life.

The infectious disease doctors recommended that I start a six-week course on an extremely potent antibiotic to be administered intravenously. The hematologist agreed but stated I couldn't take such a strong drug in my present emaciated condition. He wanted to build up my weight first.

Dr. Stewart recommended installing a central line called a triple lumen, a device he helped invent, to accomplish those goals.

The plan was to place the triple lumen in my subclavian vein under my collarbone. While only one needle entered my body, the device had three ports to insert fluids or to draw blood. Next, my body would be pumped full of weight-enhancing fluids, and then I would start the new antibiotics by i.v.

When Jack made his daily visit to see me later that day, he was alarmed to see the curtain drawn completely around my bed. When the curtain opened momentarily, one of the nurses attending to me scurried over to the medical supply area. Through that opening Jack caught a glimpse of Dr. Christianson and a resident surgeon working over my upper body. The rest of me was completely covered with green surgical sheets.

Jack was frantic. The hospital staff kept him away from my bed area but couldn't or wouldn't tell him what was going on.

During the couple of hours it took to complete the procedure (which was complicated by my artificial left shoulder), Jack told me later that his mind conjured up all sorts of complications I might have suffered, including cardiac arrest.

With the triple lumen finally in place, the doctors summoned a portable X-ray unit to make sure the device was properly installed and had not punctured my lung.

Jack was very relieved to find out what actually was going on.

As I was explaining the doctors' plan to Jack, a nurse hung a huge bag of liquid fat, called lipids, on my i.v. pole and plugged it into my new central line. Simultaneously, she started sugar water and regular saline solution into my i.v.

As the lipids started dripping into my body, I looked at Jack through my sunken, hollow eyes and said: "Now I'm on my way back. It's about time. I was starting to look like Yorick."

Jack smiled weakly at my attempt at humor, even though his concern about me was clearly etched in his face.

When Dr. Christianson showed up a short time later to check my i.v., Jack was anxious to find out more about the new antibiotic. "Are there any major side effects?" he asked.

"This can be a very dangerous drug," Dr. Christianson revealed. "It can cause hearing loss, kidney failure, low blood counts, and other complications."

"That sounds pretty scary," I opined.

"Of course, this doesn't mean that you will experience all or any of those side effects, but the potential is there," Dr. Christianson added. "We really have no choice, however. We must act quickly to turn this infection around."

Dr. Christianson explained that as soon as I started gaining some weight, they would start the new antibiotic.

Within a couple of days, my skin, wrinkled by the weight loss of the past several weeks, began to look normal again. Dr. Christianson decided it was now time to begin the six weeks of around-the-clock i.v. infusions with the antibiotic.

After a couple of weeks my weight returned to normal. Although the lipids and high calorie fluids helped me regain my weight, my cholesterol levels must have been skyrocketing off the charts.

As I gained weight, my body felt stronger. I could sense that my natural resistance—combined with the antibiotic—was gradually turning the infection around.

When my appetite returned, I began eating a high calorie diet. Jack brought me milk shakes and caramel sundaes for after-dinner snacks.

By now my weight was up to 120 pounds, an all-time high for me. Jack kidded me about my chipmunk-like cheeks.

The bedside debridement continued throughout this time.

A new surgical intern on orthopedic rotation, Dr. Malinowski, was now assigned to do the debridement and to pack and dress the open wound.

Dr. Malinowski was a blond, Polish-American from the Chicago area. Since he had taught school before coming into the Army, he was a bit older and more mature than the average intern. I was impressed by his complete professionalism.

Near the end of October, my mom returned for another visit. Jack dropped her off at the hospital on his way to work, and she normally spent the day with me.

One day during this time Dr. Malinowski came by for debridement and to change the dressing of my wound. He asked my mother if she would hold my leg straight while he was repacking it.

After Dr. Malinowski got my leg unwrapped, I noticed Mom averting her eyes to avoid having to see the bloody cavern.

When the doctor finished repacking my leg, my Mother seemed shocked. "Oh, Mary, that's the worst looking thing I've ever seen," she declared.

"The doctors seem to think it's getting a whole lot better," I reassured her.

"Do you know what it reminds me of?" she asked. Before I could answer, she replied: "The meat locker at your dad's grocery store. Your leg looks like a piece of beef on a hook!"

Periodically during the course of taking the antibiotic, the hospital staff checked me for the dreaded side effects Dr. Christianson had mentioned earlier. So far, everything seemed normal.

One day a young Hispanic audiologist came by to give me a hearing test. I thought at first he was from San Antonio, but his accent indicated he was not. He said he was from Panama. As he readied his equipment to begin the test, my mind drifted back to our experiences in Panama.

While Jack was stationed in Puerto Rico, we decided to take a week-long cruise from San Juan to Guantanamo Bay, Cuba, to Panama and return. As a military family, at that time we could go space available aboard a Military Sea Transport Service (MSTS) ship.

The ship, while not a floating luxury hotel by any means, was quite comfortable, and the other passengers were very congenial.

Our first stop, in Cuba, was interesting because the Naval Station at Guantanamo was the only American enclave in a hostile communist territory. As our ship approached the island, we were constantly shadowed by Castro's patrol boats. We had lunch there and a good visit with old Navy friends.

When our ship docked at Colon on the Atlantic side of the isthmus, we travelled by bus to Panama City on the Pacific coast. Unfortunately, the highway route didn't allow us to see much of the canal, as it passed through banana plantations and small villages in the interior of the country overrun with bare-bottomed youngsters.

In Panama City we stayed at an old Victorian-style hotel which obviously, hadn't changed any since Teddy Roosevelt's days. Our bathroom, featuring elaborate tile floors and a tub on legs, was large enough for roller skating.

Panama, a free port, in those days was a shopping paradise. I stocked up on linens, silver, filigree jewelry, and gifts from Hong Kong and other places around the globe.

In order to see more of the canal, we decided to return to our ship in Colon via the Panama Railroad. Originally built in 1850, the railway was rebuilt during construction of the canal. When we boarded the quaint, open-windowed passenger car, it was apparent that nothing had changed since 1902. The train was powered by either a wood- or coal-burning steam engine.

We had just settled in for the two-hour, 48-mile trip when I stuck my head out the window to get a better view of the Pacific Ocean fading away from us in the distance.

Suddenly, a large cinder from the engine struck my right eye and lodged securely under my lid. The pain was not as intense as it was constant.

Jack immediately tried to remove the cinder, but it was so deeply imbedded he couldn't see it. After Jack had worked over me for about fifteen minutes, the conductor and several Panamanian passengers also joined the first aid effort.

Nothing worked.

By now my eye was so irritated that I had to keep it closed all the time. That, in turn, caused my left eye to water, and I could only open it half way.

As we passed the engineering marvels—the famous Panama Canal locks—containing huge ships from all parts of the world, I could only sit in frustration with one eye closed and the other half open.

Finally, as our train pulled into the terminal at Colon, I opened both eyes, and the cinder popped out just as mysteriously as it had landed there originally.

As we boarded our ship, Jack looked at me and smiled. "Nothing simple ever happens to you, does it?" he asked.

"I guess not, Jack," I replied. "But it might have been worse. I could have caught malaria instead of a cinder."

Chapter Thirty-Six

The audiology test revealed I had not yet suffered any hearing loss from the antibiotic.

Dr. Malinowski continued to debride and repack my wound every couple of days as the antibiotic gradually seemed to be gaining on the infection.

Since he was also teaching a class of hospital corpsmen, Dr. Malinowski asked if he could show the class my wound the next time he dressed my leg. He felt my leg was probably as close to a battlefield wound as a lot of the students would ever see short of another war.

"Fine," I agreed. "I might as well earn my keep."

A couple of days later, Dr. Malinowski escorted in about a dozen fresh-faced corpsmen. As he went about his normal routine of opening the wound and removing the packing, one of the corpsmen got paler each minute. Finally, he fainted dead away.

One of the corpsman's fellow students ran for some smelling salts and revived him.

I heard later on the grapevine that the young man changed his specialty from hospital corpsman to pay clerk.

I had now been in the hospital for almost three and a half months. Every recent culture taken from my leg came back negative for *Pseudomonas*. Jack was about at his wits end trying to juggle his busy schedule. I decided it was time to find a way for me to go home.

That evening after rounds Dr. Bucknell and Dr. Christianson stayed on to talk with me. I wanted to know their master plan.

"I can't stay here and vegetate forever," I began. "What are we going to do with my leg?"

"We would like to put in a rod to replace your femur," Dr. Bucknell revealed. "But we can't do that now for fear of reintroducing the infection. We might let you go home if Jack could do for you there what we are doing here."

"Do you think Jack could dress your wound at home, Mary?" Dr. Christianson asked.

"That's asking a lot of Jack. He's good at a lot of things. If it were for a third party, I'm sure he could," I said. "But I don't think he could pull out the packing, repack the wound, and change bandages on someone he loved. He would be too emotionally involved and afraid he was hurting me."

The same conversation resumed the next evening with the two doctors. This time, after 24 hours of reflection, I was more forceful.

After several minutes of talking I finally said what was on my mind. "There are a lot of things in life worse than not being able to walk. I still have one leg. Maybe in six months we can regroup. Let me get home," I pleaded. "Let's take my leg out of traction. Let's just sew it up and leave it the way it is."

Orthopedic doctors don't like to hear that kind of talk. They want patients to leave in better shape than they arrived. They looked stunned. "Do you know what that would entail?" Dr. Bucknell finally asked. "Your leg will shrink. You'll never be able to bear any weight on it."

"I know. But I can use crutches. I can use a wheelchair part of the time. Our new home is all on one level. I've got to get out of the hospital. I've got to get on with my life."

After several more points and counterpoints, the doctors reluctantly agreed to my request. As Dr. Bucknell departed, he said he would schedule the surgery to close my leg.

About an hour later, Dr. Christianson returned. "Dr. Bucknell and I were talking some more about your case, Mary," he began. "We wanted you to know you have another option other than just sewing up your leg."

"What is it?"

"Well, we could amputate it."

I was surprised. I had always thought of amputation as a last resort. "Oh, I don't know, I've kind of become attached to this leg," I joked. "At least it will fill out the other side of my slacks."

In a more serious vein, I asked: "Is there any medical reason to amputate?"

"No. And we really don't want to," Dr. Christianson added. "Orthopedic doctors don't like to throw away good bone. And you've got good bone from the knee down."

"Then let's go ahead and sew it up," I suggested.

I was placed on the operating schedule for two days later.

By now we were nearing the middle of November, and I was becoming concerned that I might not make it home for Thanksgiving. About a month earlier I had wagered a turkey with one of the orthopedic residents, Dr. Cruz, that I would be home by Thanksgiving.

When I rolled into the operating room for the fourteenth time since August, I saw Dr. Bucknell and Dr. Christianson in their scrubs. "Guys, do you think I'll make it home for Thanksgiving?"

"For sure!" Dr. Bucknell stated emphatically.

"Okay, you tell Dr. Cruz the next time you see him that he owes me a turkey if I get out of here."

Both doctors chuckled as the anesthesiologist put me to sleep.

The next time I woke up I had been moved out of isolation and back to the regular part of the ward. After almost three months in quarantine, it was great to be back with "real" people again.

The next morning Dr. Bucknell removed my bandage to change it, and I caught my first look at my leg after surgery. Since the wound had been open so long, they couldn't use traditional suture methods to close it. Instead, the outer skin was closed loosely with the threads circling through marshmallow-like anchors. This technique also was designed to promote healing from inside out.

It was now time to begin physical therapy in earnest. During my months of hospitalization, Ben Gallegos, one of the PT corpsmen, worked with me as much as possible considering I was confined to bed with one leg in traction. But now it was time to prepare me to use crutches and to transfer to wheelchairs.

Since I had been lying on my back for so long, the therapists decided I'd better start sitting up in small doses. The next morning after surgery, Ben rolled in a lounge chair and parked it next to my bed. "When we transfer you over to this chair you'll feel light-headed, Mrs. Walker," Ben explained. "Just let us know when you want to go back to bed."

Ben lifted me over to the chair at 10 a.m. Since I didn't call to ask to return to bed, Ben came back in about an hour to check on me. "Want to go back to bed?"

"No, Ben, I'm doing fine. I want to wait until Jack comes in at noon."

About an hour later when Jack showed up, he was so surprised to see me sitting in a chair I thought he was going to faint.

All he could do was kiss me and shake his head in disbelief.

I smiled at him and said exuberantly: "Honey, I'm on my way back! Today sitting up! Tomorrow, crutches!"

Sitting in a chair after almost four months in a hospital bed and using crutches are two different challenges. Therefore, we progressed a bit more slowly to crutches.

My incision continued to drain a great deal even though there were no tubes. It was not uncommon to soak through a bandage in 24 hours. Dr. Malinowski reassured me that this was normal and urged me not to be alarmed.

Each time Ben or one of the other therapists got me up to

practice with crutches, it seemed my bandage fell off. Finally, we all concluded that my incision was a very difficult place to make a bandage secure.

To help remedy the situation, the next day Dr. Malinowski brought some surgical net, which is often used around a person's abdomen after general surgery, to put on my leg and hold the bandage in place.

"This is crummy," I teased. "If I have to wear this surgical net on my leg, it should at least be a sexy color. This hospital white is no turn on."

A couple of days later, Dr. Malinowski returned with a red net (dyed with iodine, no doubt) to replace the white one.

From then on, I walked around the hospital on crutches with my sexy red net showing beneath my gown.

Each day I extended my walking distance on crutches as I felt my strength slowly returning. Dr. Bucknell was right, however, because in the short time which elapsed since my final surgery, I could feel my leg was indeed shrinking.

The wound continued to drain as well and probably would for several more weeks, according to the doctors.

In order for me to go home, Jack needed to learn how to clean the incision and change the dressing and bandages daily using sterile conditions. Dr. Malinowski gave him the short course and, being a quick learn, Jack declared he was ready for me to come home.

After almost four months in the hospital, the doctors said I could go home the day before Thanksgiving.

The physical therapy gang baked a cake, and the entire staff held a big celebration for me on the ward. When I left, I hugged and kissed everyone goodbye. To just say "thanks" for all they had done for me seemed so inadequate. But for now, that would have to suffice.

Oddly enough, I really felt sad leaving. In a way it was like leaving my extended family. But I was ecstatic to be able to go home to my real family once again.

The next day Jack's sister, Kay, invited us and the other local relatives over for Thanksgiving dinner. It was truly a day to give thanks.

The only shoes I could get my feet into after such a long time was a pair of moccasins.

When I crutched into Kay's house, Jack's niece, Debbie, looked at me, laughed, and said: "Aunt Mary, it's wonderful that you came in moccasins to represent the Indian contingent who were at the first Thanksgiving."

As we all had a good laugh, I knew at long last I was finally home.

Chapter Thirty-Seven

"Well, how does it smell?" I asked Jack as he sniffed my bandage during his daily ritual of dressing my incision.

"Real good," he assured me, which meant that he didn't detect any infectious odor.

Jack had become quite adept at this chore since I came home from the hospital. In fact, I've always thought that he would have been an excellent physician. He certainly was intelligent enough. But, more importantly, he had a great bedside manner and an abundance of empathy for anyone with a medical problem.

We were now well into December, and our house remained unsold. Each month, several prospective buyers looked at it, but the right person had not yet materialized.

As Christmas neared, we transformed our home with decorations acquired from years of traveling and living in exotic places. Of course, as always, a natural tree stood majestically in a corner of the family room, radiating the unique fragrance of Christmas. The smell of fresh-baked Christmas cookies and cakes blended with the aroma of fir to produce a warm, homey ambiance.

If the house was to be shown when I was gone, I always left a plate of fresh-baked cookies with a note explaining my absence and urging the visitors to help themselves to the cookies.

Either through a combination of my baking, the holiday spirit, or just plain luck, our real estate agent called about a week before Christmas with a contract on our house. Although the offering price was somewhat less than we were asking, we accepted the bid without a counter proposal. After almost nine months on the market, our house finally sold.

We closed on our San Antonio house and moved into our new home on Valentine's Day, 1986.

Once we had the move behind us and got settled, we felt like we had acquired a little piece of heaven.

Both our children opted to stay in the city to work until college started the next fall. So it was just Jack and I in our dream home with Snoopy and Loki (a Siamese cat we had acquired three years earlier) together with our three horses who had been holding down our 40 acres until we moved out to join them.

From our gorgeous hilltop, we had unobstructed views of the ever-changing palette of the Texas sunsets. Herds of deer grazed in our valley while squirrels, and birds of every hue, played in our trees. Armadillos, raccoons, and opossum were our constant nocturnal neighbors.

As soon as we were settled enough to do so, we invited all the physicians, nurses, corpsmen, and staff who had waited on me for those four months to join us in a series of open houses. One LVN who had been in the medical profession for over 40 years said this was the first time a patient ever really followed through and gave such an event.

Professionally, the orthopedic doctors continued to keep a close watch on my leg. Finally, in late March, the seeping from my wound stopped, and we no longer needed to keep it bandaged.

A month later, while visiting the dermatologist about removing a wart on my finger, the doctor found another suspicious-looking spot on my back. Sure enough, a shave biopsy revealed the presence of basal skin cancer again. Since my treatment in 1984 cured me of this type of cancer before, I was confident that modern medicine could do the same thing again. After minor surgery, my skin returned to normal quickly.

Later that summer while Jack and I were returning from a visit to Georgetown, we stopped at The University of Texas while we were in Austin. Ever since my recovery from the infection, I had been pestering Jack about going to UT football games again. He wasn't sure what accommodations, if any, there were for fans in wheelchairs. The last game we attended I had to climb on crutches to the top row of the upper deck to reach our seat. When the box office attendant assured us they had up-to-date wheelchair facilities, we purchased tickets for the first home game that fall.

When we arrived at Memorial Stadium and rolled into the wheelchair section, we couldn't believe our good fortune. Our seats were right up next to the press box under a covered area with protection from rain and, in Texas, particularly important, from the blistering sun of early fall. The seats were high enough to give us an excellent view of the entire field, but not so elevated as to obscure important details.

My wheelchair was parked perpendicular to a long counter in front of me, high enough above the row below me that even when the fans stood, I could still see all parts of the field. Jack sat on a raised stool behind me as my "attendant."

Standing in the south end zone was the University's mascot, Bevo, a Texas longhorn, signifying the spirit of the great State of Texas. This magnificent burnt orange and white animal, now relatively docile after years of domestication, was a direct descendant from those wild-tough monarchs of the Texas plains of the last century able to survive all adversaries, including the harsh weather, where others would surely perish.

On our way home I was still enraptured by all the pageantry and excitement of big-time college football. When I asked Jack about buying season tickets for the rest of that year, he agreed. "But there's something wrong with the system," he laughed. "I have to take my Midwestern-born, handicapped wife to my alma mater to get decent seats at the football games."

I tease Jack often when we go to other sports events at UT that if he happens to cross me, I may end up taking another attendant.

With our empty nest, we also now were free to subscribe to both the Houston Grand Opera and The Dallas Operas. We had attended individual performances at both houses in the past, but not as subscribers.

Snoopy, our faithful pet of fifteen years, began to deteriorate dramatically during the fall of 1986. Initially, she lost any semblance of her former voracious appetite. As she lost weight, she became weaker. Then both her liver and kidneys failed. Finally, she was too weak to walk, and Jack had to carry her skeleton-like body from place to place.

Reluctantly, with no quality of life remaining, we were forced to follow our veterinarian's advice to put her to sleep.

Jack carried Snoopy into the doctor's office and gently placed her on the treatment table. Her hollow, brown eyes, normally sad looking even in times of good health, looked up at us imploringly. "What," she seemed to be asking us, "has happened to me?"

All of us wept uncontrollably as the vet injected the vial of life-ending drug into her vein. Within seconds, Snoopy died peacefully and quietly without any evidence of pain or trauma.

After living with us for fifteen years, Snoopy's death was almost like losing a child. Both Jack and I agreed that Snoopy would be our last dog. It was far too difficult to go through that experience again.

During the early part of 1987, I experienced some strange episodes where my heart would seem to skip beats or palpitate unpredictably.

When my oncologist sent me to cardiology, I was seen by Dr. Wellford, a slight, youthful-looking man in his early thirties. He gave me several tests, including a treadmill (done by turning a wheel with my arms), an echogram, another MUGA scan, and a thalium test.

After all the results were in, I saw Dr. Wellford again in April.

"Mrs. Walker," the doctor began, "I have some good news and some bad news."

"Let's have the good news first," I suggested.

"Okay. Your cholesterol count is pretty good for a wheelchair person."

When I told him about being able to swim a quarter of a mile a day in our indoor pool, he seemed pleased about me getting that much exercise.

"What's the bad news?" I asked.

"Somewhere along the way you've had a silent heart attack which has damaged your heart muscle quite a bit."

I was shocked. I couldn't recall experiencing any chest pains or heart irregularities which could even remotely approximate the extreme pain normally associated with a heart attack.

Dr. Wellford placed me on a strict, low-fat, low-cholesterol diet along with some heart medication and the advice to get as much exercise as I could.

Why I suffered the attack may never be known. Jack and I speculated that the continued toxicity of Adriamycin, combined with all the lipids pumped into my bloodstream during my recovery from the infection, may have been the cause. In any case, there is little doubt that my heart problems were the direct result of having cancer.

Jack decided earlier that year that he needed a Wagner "fix," as he called his desire from time to time to attend one of the German composer's works. So he chose the largest fix of all with *Der Ring Des Nibelungen*, to be held in Seattle in August.

Since my heart seemed to have settled down some, Jack thought it was time for me to take the plunge as well. Although I knew a lot of the music from recordings, I had never seen the complete *Ring* in person.

When we returned to our hotel after the opening night production of *Das Rheingold*, a message to call home awaited us. Amy tearfully told us she was involved in an accident and had totalled our pickup truck. As soon as we determined she miraculously escaped unhurt, we decided to stay the rest of the week for the other three music dramas of Wagner's tetralogy.

Since I had been to Seattle years earlier with the Aqua Follies, I had the rare opportunity to act as tour guide for Jack. Between performances, we visited old Navy friends, took in Seattle and its environs, and made a boat trip to Victoria, British Columbia, including a visit to the magnificent Butchart Gardens.

After the thrilling finale of *Götterdämmerung*, I could tell from Jack's beatific expression that he had obtained his fix. But after almost sixteen hours of Wagner's music, I felt like my posterior was "fixed" to my wheelchair.

Shortly after returning home, I reported to the gynecologist for my routine annual pap smear. During the examination, the doctor discovered blood in my stool sample. With my medical history, such a discovery always sends up a red flag in the minds of medical people.

Consequently, I was dispatched to general surgery for a proctoscope exam which turned out negative. To be on the safe side, they followed up with a barium enema. However, because I couldn't stand up, it was impossible to get a good picture. Since my tests thus far were either negative or inconclusive, the surgeons decided prudence required that I undergo a colonoscopy. I was sent home and told I would be contacted by the surgeon who was to perform the exam.

A couple of days later I answered my phone and heard a male voice. "Mrs. Walker, this is Dr. Olson from general surgery. I'd like to schedule your colonoscopy."

"Not the Dr. Olson who called me back to the hospital from my weekend pass in 1985?" I asked.

"That depends. Is this the Mrs. Walker I knew on the orthopedic ward?" Dr. Olson responded.

"It sure is," I affirmed. "But I thought you were going to be an orthopedic surgeon."

"After my association with you, I decided that general surgery was where I wanted to be," he bantered. "Besides, I'm so good at doing colonoscopies that people come from miles around to have me perform it."

The Fat Lady Hasn't Sung

I was looking forward to seeing Dr. Olson again as I was wheeled into the examining room. Although a nurse gave me some Valium, I was wide awake when Dr. Olson and his colleague began their exploration. As they carefully looked inside my colon, I engaged them in conversation ranging from the weather to sports.

When the doctors completed the examination, since I was so wide awake and involved in their activities, Dr. Olson asked if I'd like to see inside my colon.

Naturally, I jumped at the opportunity. It was at once a wonderful but eerie experience to travel through one's own intestinal tract via the wizardry of modern medicine. It was like being inside a huge worm.

A few days later I received the results of the colonoscopy: "within normal limits; no evidence of malignancy."

Of course, Jack and I were overjoyed by my dodging another bullet. After such exhaustive testing and coming up negative, the source of the original blood would have to remain still another of life's mysteries.

Amy decided to transfer to the University of North Texas, about 300 miles north of San Antonio in Denton, beginning with the fall semester. So in late August, Amy and her dad loaded our car to the ceiling, and in Okie-like fashion, we set out on our long hot trek. Naturally, Amy's dormitory room was on the third floor. Poor Jack must have made a hundred trips up those stairs carrying enough clothes to supply the whole dorm.

After our trip to Denton, we were looking forward to a nice, relaxing Labor Day weekend.

As we got ready for bed Saturday night, Jack pushed me back to our bedroom as usual in my companion chair—a chair similar to a regular chair except it has small wheels at the base of each of its four legs. I was carrying a pile of clean clothes I had washed earlier.

When Jack took some towels into the bathroom, I thought I would make myself useful and push with my feet across the room to put away our underwear.

As I started across the carpet, one of the small wheels must have caught in the plush thickness. The next thing I knew, I was lying face down on the floor of our bedroom with the companion chair folded up next to me.

Jack raced in from the bathroom as soon as he heard the noise. "What have you done?" he shouted anxiously. "Let me help you up!"

"Please don't touch me," I cautioned him. "I'm just in agony! Just let me lie here for a bit," I pleaded. "Oh, Jack, I think I've done something really bad!"

Jack looked bewildered. He wanted to help but didn't know what to do. "Is it your shoulder?" he asked, concerned that I may have damaged my prosthesis.

"Oh, no, that isn't what hurts. It's my right leg. I think it's broken."

After lying on the floor for a few more moments, I realized I had to do something. "If you could pull on my leg, maybe I could roll over on my back."

Jack wasn't too keen about my suggestion. "I can't pull on your leg. I might make it worse."

"Just act like you are traction," I instructed him. "Pull slowly but firmly."

Jack followed my directions reluctantly. As he pulled my leg, I slowly rolled over on my back.

After adjusting to my new position for a moment, I said, "Now this doesn't feel so bad. I'll just lie here for a little while."

"I'm calling EMS," Jack said as he headed for the phone.

"Oh, Jack, please don't. We can't have someone come out here this late," I pleaded. By now it was past midnight.

"For heaven's sake, Mary! That's their job."

"No, I'll just lie here on the floor until morning," I suggested as I got more comfortable. "Just get me a pillow, and cover me with a blanket."

Jack was exasperated. I'm sure he thought I must have cracked my head in the fall the way I was resisting outside help.

I finally convinced him we weren't going to bother EMS.

"Well, can't I pick you up?" he suggested.

When I said no, he had another idea. "Maybe we can devise something to at least get you into bed."

My silence was Jack's signal to begin rigging up a splint which he slid under my right leg and secured with some belts. With his help, I was then able to transfer from the floor to a low footstool. Then from the footstool he placed my transfer board up to the bed. I slowly pulled myself up the incline as Jack steadied my leg much like going up a slide backwards.

After almost a half hour of struggling, I finally flopped onto the bed.

Jack removed the splint as I tried to maneuver myself into a comfortable position. "It really doesn't feel too bad now," I said. "I think I'll be all right. If you would get me a Valium, I'll just wait until morning."

"If you won't call EMS, would you please call the hospital?" Jack begged. "Please just see what the doctor says."

I finally acquiesced to Jack's pleas. It was now almost 2 a.m. by the time I got through to the on-call orthopedic doctor.

Dr. Wiggins, a new resident, listened politely as I told him about my fall and the subsequent pain in my leg. When I finished talking, he was reassuring. "I don't think you've broken your femur, Mrs. Walker. That's the longest bone in your body. It takes an awful lot to break it, especially for someone as young as you. You've probably just pulled some muscles. But if it's still bothering you in the morning, come in."

Jack was totally frustrated. I wouldn't let him call EMS, and now the orthopedic doctor seemed to play down my situation. Reluctantly, Jack brought me some Valium and a couple of Tylenol pills which Dr. Wiggins had recommended.

I slept the rest of the night like a baby while poor Jack lay awake beside me worrying.

At 7:30 he woke me saying we had to get to the hospital, and he was calling EMS.

Within fifteen minutes, two young paramedics arrived. I told them about my fall eight hours earlier and that I may have broken my femur.

They both seemed to indulge my view of my injury as they busily splinted my leg and lifted me onto a gurney. They didn't bother to start an i.v. or splint my leg properly as required by EMS regulations in situations of suspected bone fracture. Both men thought I didn't have enough pain for a broken leg. Like the doctor, they thought I had pulled muscles.

When I arrived at the BAMC emergency room after chatting with the EMS technicians during the entire 30-mile trip, I had to wait a while to be seen by a doctor, who immediately ordered X-rays.

About two hours after my arrival, a technician brought in an envelope containing my newest films.

"Well, is it broken?" I asked.

"I can't comment on things like that," he replied. "You'll have to talk to the doctor."

"Oh, come on," I pleaded. "You've seen hundreds of X-rays. Surely you would know."

"Okay, Mrs. Walker, I'll let *you* look at it," he agreed, as he handed me one of the films.

As I held the X-ray up to the light, it was like 1985 all over again.

There in the black and white images I saw my right femur bone with a compound fracture in the identical spot where my left thigh was broken two years earlier.

Chapter Thirty-Eight

The emergency room doctor of the day, Dr. Du Jour, as he jokingly introduced himself, confirmed my unofficial diagnosis: my right femur was fractured.

In short order I was loaded aboard an Army ambulance for the mile or so trip to the orthopedic ward at Beach Pavilion.

As soon as we turned the first corner, my gurney scooted across the deck of the rear compartment of the ambulance and careened off the adjacent wall. At the next corner, I shot back the other way, crashing into the opposite wall. I was starting to feel like a handball.

I finally maneuvered the gurney into a position where I could knock on the window between me and the driver. As soon as I got his attention, he stopped immediately and ran around to the back of the vehicle, apologizing profusely for failing to secure my gurney properly.

As he locked the wheels and strapped me to the wall, I tried to put him at ease. "For a moment, I thought I might have to be hospitalized not just with a broken leg, but also with head injuries."

When I arrived at the orthopedic ward, I was met by Dr. Behrens, a new resident who by now had relieved Dr. Wiggins of the ward duty.

"It looks like you've really done a job on yourself," Dr. Behrens commented as he busily supervised a technician who was placing my leg in traction.

I agreed. "But I can't stay in here very long," I added as Dr. Behrens looked puzzled. "I have to be out of here by Saturday so Jack and I can use our new-season tickets to go see our beloved Longhorns play their first home game."

"I don't know about that. I'll have to take it up with 'the man,'" Dr. Behrens replied, using the appellation the new group of residents had dubbed Dr. Bucknell.

Dr. Behrens explained that since this was Labor Day weekend, there wasn't much he could do until Tuesday when Dr. Bucknell returned except to keep me comfortable.

I took a liking to Dr. Behrens immediately. I quickly discovered that the blond Midwesterner from South Dakota was a good listener who was sensitive to the needs of his patients.

Returning to the orthopedic ward after my lengthy stay two years earlier was like old home week. Several of the nurses, LVN's, and corpsmen I had known from my previous stay welcomed me like family.

The first staff person to greet me was Julian Torres, a civilian corpsman who had once served as an Army medic and currently was studying nursing at Jack's college while working at BAMC.

We reminisced about my lengthy stay on the ward during 1985.

While I was taking all those fluids intravenously through my triple lumen, I needed a bed pan quite frequently.

During a night shift when Julian was the only corpsman on duty, I rang for a bed pan. "I'll be right there," Julian replied.

Before he could get to me, he was waylaid by an emergency and apparently forgot about me for awhile.

In the meantime, I couldn't wait any longer. I first filled my embicin basin and then started on some paper cups at my bedside.

By the time Julian finally arrived, I had filled everything around me with urine. In addition, I had spilled some on my sheets.

Two years later, that incident struck us both as funny.

"I promise you, Mary, this time I'll get your bedpans to you sooner."

"Don't worry about that anymore," I assured him. "During the past couple of years I've learned to use a male urinal. I'll just hang it on the side of my bed where I can use it when I need it, and you can empty it when you get a chance."

Julian shook his head in disbelief and chuckled.

In fact, he laughed every time he came near me since he said he wasn't used to seeing a male urinal hanging on a bed in a female ward.

Early Tuesday morning, Dr. Bucknell, accompanied by Dr. Behrens and an entourage of orthopedic residents, showed up at my bedside.

"I see you've done exactly what I warned you not to do," Dr. Bucknell chastised me gently. "I said you could do anything you want, except just don't fall."

"I know this is bad, Dr. Bucknell. But Jack and I have been thinking about my situation. I really feel the only course of action is to just remove my right femur as we did on the left."

Dr. Bucknell listened unemotionally as Dr. Behrens and the other residents seemed horrified by my words. "I don't want to go through a revision and all that. I can't walk anyway. I think it's best to just remove the bone. Besides I need to get out of here so I can go to UT's first home football game."

The doctors stood silently for a while looking at each other. Finally, Dr. Behrens spoke. "We can't do that. You'll be exactly like a squid."

Everyone laughed except Dr. Behrens. Not having lived through the nearly-catastrophic episode involving my left leg two years earlier, he was eager to pursue an orthopedic surgeon's goal of making people better, not worse, from a mobility standpoint.

Dr. Bucknell ended the discussion by announcing the staff would meet later to decide what to do.

Sure enough, on Wednesday afternoon Dr. Bucknell and his orthopedic brain trust gathered around my bed.

"After thoroughly examining your X-rays and extensive discussion, none of us are sure of the exact condition of your right femur bone, other than its being fractured," Dr. Bucknell explained. "Since that wasn't the site of the massive malignancy, the right bone may not be as bad as your left bone was."

"So you think there's a chance to save it?" I wondered.

"We think it would be wise to cast your leg and see if there isn't enough good bone left to mend eventually. At least that way you would have one leg to make transferring easier and to crutch short distances."

I was more anxious than anyone to retain as much mobility as I could. So I seized this slender reed of hope with enthusiasm. "Great! Let's do that if you think it might work." Then, with a grin, I added "Just so I get out of here by Friday so I can go to the game."

The men in the white coats surrounding my bed all laughed. "Mrs. Walker, the Longhorns won't win whether you go or not," one of the young residents teased me.

"You never know," I predicted. "I might make a difference." I seemed to be the primary focus of attention in the cast room on Friday as Dr. Bucknell supervised the efforts of a couple of residents and two or three corpsmen.

As the cast took shape, Dr. Bucknell revealed his master plan: wear the cast for six to eight weeks with periodic X-rays to determine how the healing was progressing.

When the orthopedic sculptors had finished, the cast extended from my ankle up to my groin. It then continued up my right side and wrapped around my waist like a belt, entombing my entire right side. There was no way to bend my knee or hip, and I had to sit with my leg sticking straight out.

With my cast now in place, Dr. Bucknell decided there was no further need for me to stay in the hospital and signed my discharge order.

So that I could get home without having to wear my hospital garb, Jack brought along a large pair of his shorts which I could pull on over my cast.

Even though Jack was delighted to have me home again, he was apprehensive about us going to the game the next day. I finally convinced him that with such a massive cast, I couldn't move my leg whether I was at home or anywhere else. Therefore, there was no reason not to go.

With Jack's help, I put on one of my larger pants suits, and we were on our way to Austin on Saturday afternoon. (Due to the late summer heat, the first couple of home games are always played in the evening).

We arrived at Memorial Stadium about an hour before kickoff, and I went directly to the rest room. Once in the handicapped stall, I struggled for several minutes trying to get my slacks down over my cast. I finally won the tug-of-war and emptied my bladder.

But getting my pants down and pulling them back up proved to be two different challenges. I pulled and tussled and struggled to no avail. Something on the cast was binding. I glanced at my watch and noticed it was getting close to kickoff time as I renewed my efforts. Thoughts of spending part or all of the game in the ladies' room trying to pull up my pants raced through my mind.

No matter how hard I fought, the pants wouldn't budge.

Finally, in desperation, I pulled my shirt down as far as possible to cover up anything that might be visible and wheeled out to where Jack was waiting, literally with my fanny completely uncovered.

"What in the world has taken you so long?" Jack asked nervously.

"My slacks are binding! I can't pull them up."

Jack laughed when he saw my predicament. "You're out here mooning everybody," he teased as he began to help. "We'll make it fit," he vowed as he pulled and tugged.

By now we were beginning to attract attention from some of the late-arriving fans.

As Jack gave a stronger than usual jerk, the material finally tore, and he pulled my slacks up to their normal position.

"You *made* it fit all right," I agreed.

As Jack pushed me to our seats, the Longhorn band already was playing "The Star-Spangled Banner."

"It's a shame we aren't playing Miami instead of BYU tonight," Jack observed.

"Why?"

"You would have fit right in as the 'moon over Miami,'" he joked as we settled in to watch the game.

Four weeks later I reported back to the orthopedic clinic as instructed. Dr. Behrens, either through wishful thinking or scientific evidence, thought he saw some signs of the bone healing. Now, however, instead of six weeks in the cast, it definitely would be eight.

Fortunately, after my ordeal at the football game, I acquired some new skirts, thus eliminating my constant struggle with pulling my slacks over my cast.

Of course, as long as I was cast bound, there was no way I could swim. I convinced Jack he should continue his daily swimming routine even though I wasn't doing laps with him. I did serve as his lifeguard, with the cleaning pole in readiness in case of an emergency.

When eight weeks finally passed, I went back to orthopedics again for X-rays.

As Dr. Behrens studied the images, I made small talk about the difficulties of living in a cast for two months. "I sure will be glad to get rid of this cast! You should see how I've skinned up my wooden chairs at home."

Dr. Behrens remained silent as he continued to gaze at the lighted screen. Finally, he looked at me dejectedly. "Mary, it isn't healing."

"I can't believe it," I replied. "I've had this cast on for two months! How about my other joints? Wearing this cast can't be good for them. How much longer?"

"Let's try it another month," Dr. Behrens suggested. "If it hasn't healed by then, we'll have to try something else."

Reluctantly I agreed, not that I had many choices.

When I got home, I transferred to a lounge chair and elevated my feet. I looked at my toes, swollen from weeks of being in a cast. It brought back memories of the first time I had a cast on my leg when we were living on Guam.

From 1969 to 1971 Jack was the Executive Officer at the Naval Communication Station on Guam. With 70 officers and 1700 enlisted personnel in the command, Jack worked long, irregular hours. In spite of the demands of his job, we all enjoyed our stay on the island where "America's day begins."

Our quarters backed right up to the jungle—a tropical growth so dense that we were always somewhat wary about what might come out of there someday. Jack told us about the "last" Japanese soldier hold out from World War II (who didn't know that the war had been over for more than 20 years) came out of the Guam jungle a few years before we arrived.

As we gazed out our dining room window, Jack often jested with us about being alert for any more World War II stragglers.

(In 1972, about a year after returning to Washington, D.C., we read in the newspaper about yet another Japanese soldier from World War II, Sgt. Shoichi Yokoi, who had somehow survived nearly 28 years undetected in the jungles of Guam. He didn't know the war was over.)

We never saw any strange humans come out of the jungle, but we did see a variety of exotic wildlife.

Wild pigs playfully danced around the edges of the tropical undergrowth at dusk. A pair of large monitor lizards occasionally scurried in and out of the foliage, their spiny-ridged backs making them look like throwbacks to the dinosaur age. I told David and Amy they were probably husband and wife.

Our residence, built by Navy Seabees, was a long rambler with a front door and two side doors. Our kids and their friends used all three doors constantly, sometimes failing to close them securely.

One day as I was cleaning our bedroom, I walked around our bed and came eye to eye with an enormous lizard, standing there as if it were the master of the house.

I was so shocked and frightened that I ran out of the room, slamming the door shut behind me. "Amy, stand guard at the door!" I shouted as I dashed to the phone to call Jack.

As usual, I caught Jack at a bad time. "You've got to come home!" I pleaded, trying to explain the creature in our bedroom.

"Mary, I'm so busy I don't know if I can come home right now. Are you sure it isn't one of those green geckos?"

"This lizard is so big I could saddle it up and let Amy ride it out. Please come home!"

When Jack arrived, the four of us, plus David's friend, marched down the hall toward our prey.

Of course, when Jack opened the door, the lizard was nowhere to be seen. We looked in the closets; we moved furniture out from the wall; we pulled dresses out of the closets and looked behind them. There were no uninvited guests to be seen.

Finally, Jack gave instructions to David. "Lie down and see if you can see it under our bed."

David followed his Dad's directions. "Yep. He's under there," David replied unemotionally as if we had a large lizard under our bed every day of the week.

Amy, by contrast, was now standing on top of our dresser.

Jack bent down to confirm the lizard's presence, still thinking I might have overreacted. I was vindicated by what he saw: a three-foot long monitor lizard sticking out its tongue at him.

Using a broom and a garden rake, Jack herded the reptile toward the side door. Each time it got near the threshold, it clawed and fought to stay in the house. Finally, Jack pushed it out the door, and it scurried off toward the jungle.

Thereafter, every time we saw the pair of lizards near the jungle's edge, we knew they were happy to be reunited. But they couldn't be nearly as happy as we were to have the beast out from under our bed.

A few weeks later while I was ironing, Amy ran up to me excitedly and exclaimed: "Mommy, Mommy! There's a lizard in the house!"

I followed her to the living room, thinking surely we can't have another monitor lizard inside. Sure enough, it was a little green gecko.

In an effort to catch it to let it outside, I tried to step on its tail. Instead, I turned my ankle and fell on the tile floor. A sharp pain shot through my foot and leg. I lay on the floor for a while staring at the ceiling. "Now what have I done?" I thought. "What a klutz!"

Amy, who was only about two and a half years old, wanted to help me so I instructed her on how to dial the phone. After she dialed Jack's number, Amy's little voice said to his secretary: "I want to talk to my Daddy." After a few seconds, she spoke again. "Mommy's hurt. Daddy, come home."

Amy hung up the phone and came over to lie down beside me to await Jack. Meanwhile, David and his friend came in, looked at me on the floor, and asked if he and Bruce could have something to drink. He was so casual about the whole situation that one might conclude he saw me lying on the floor everyday.

Within minutes of Amy's call, Jack was home helping me up. He carried me to the car, loaded up the kids, and we all set out for the hospital.

Predictably, with the pain I was experiencing along with the swelling, I had broken a small bone in my foot.

To pay for my folly, I had to wear a leg cast for eight weeks in Guam's heat and humidity.

As I sat in my chair in Texas, I thought how nice it would be to be back on Guam even chasing lizards instead of wearing this half-body cast for three months.

Chapter Thirty-Nine

One month to the day I was back in the Orthopedic Clinic again with fresh X-rays and the hope that after three months I might be able to shed my cumbersome cast.

"You know, Mary, it looks like some mending might be taking place," Dr. Behrens stated optimistically as he gazed at the new films. "In any case, we're going to take your cast off and put you in a removable foam and velcro stabilizer. That way you can take it off to wash and bathe."

"What about swimming?"

"No swimming. Your bone is just starting to knit. I don't want you kicking your leg in the pool. Let's give the soft cast a try, and I'll see you after the Christmas holidays."

The new cast simplified my life considerably. My foot was free so I could wear both shoes again, and I now could bend my knee with caution. But being able to shower again was the biggest treat of all.

When I returned to the clinic in mid-January, Dr. Behrens and Dr. Bucknell concluded that there was no healing taking place beyond the initial tentative fusion.

I was disappointed but not surprised.

Having apparently determined that my right femur would never heal, Dr. Bucknell recommended that I check into the hospital to prepare for the inevitable surgery to remove the bone.

After completing my pre-operative tests, a visitor from my past came by to see me.

Dr. Christianson was back in town on business and heard I was in the hospital again. As we visited, he reminded me of what I and everyone else went through in 1985 with *pseudomonas*. "With more surgery, there's always the possibility the infection could return," he cautioned.

As an alternative to surgery, Dr. Christianson suggested a rather radical option: take off the soft cast and learn to live with the broken bone.

"Your body will build up cartilage around the broken ends. You'll get used to it," he predicted. "You'd be like a wild animal."

As Dr. Christianson talked, I was reminded of a deer Jack and I had seen recently on our property. Although the bone in her front leg was clearly broken, she could hobble around and even run when necessary.

"What about swimming?" I wondered again.

"No problem. You can do anything you feel like doing."

"Except walk," I reminded him.

Dr. Christianson apparently had little difficulty convincing Dr. Bucknell, who wasn't too keen either about taking the risk of operating, to postpone my surgery.

After living in a cast for almost five months, I felt remarkably lighter getting around without it.

During this time we noticed the beginning of a mildew problem with our indoor pool. The warm, humid air inside, contrasted with the colder air on the outside, was causing a tremendous condensation problem on the inside walls and glass doors.

In frustration, Jack bought wet suits for both of us on the assumption that lowering the pool temperature from the comfortable 80 degrees we prefer during the winter to a cooler 70 degrees would reduce or, hopefully, stop the interior condensation.

Without my femur bone, my left leg already had shrunk about three inches so the wet suit hung loosely on that leg. In addition, even though my suit was the smallest size available, on my small frame, it resembled a potato sack. In contrast, Jack's suit fit him like his second skin. He reminded me of James Bond in one of his underwater action movies.

Each time we entered the water to swim, the cold water rushed in under my short leg and around my neck. In seconds, what seemed by contrast to my warm groin and abdomen as frigid water rushed in my suit, sending agonizing shivers throughout my body. Since the wet suit made me more buoyant, I tended to float instead of getting under the water enough for the proper swimming action.

Even worse, every time I moved my right leg, the broken ends of my femur rubbed back and forth on each other like a severed electric cable, sending a massive shock through my leg. Even without kicking, the rocking movement of the water alone activated an electrical charge.

In theory, Jack's proposed solution to the mildew problem seemed promising. In practice, we were trying to swim in uncomfortable wet suits in water cold enough for polar bears while the interior moisture continued unabated.

Wild animals undoubtedly have more tolerance for pain than I do or, more likely, have no other recourse but to endure their terrible agony or die.

After six weeks of trying to overcome my broken femur like a denizen of the forest, I returned to the Orthopedic Clinic in late February for a more civilized solution.

I explained that the natural approach wasn't working, and the pain was overwhelming at times.

Dr. Bucknell didn't seem too surprised by my experiences and reluctantly agreed to the last available alternative: to surgically remove my right femur.

Early in March of 1988 I checked into the hospital for what I hoped would be the last surgery on my legs.

When I arrived in the OR, I chatted with Dr. Bucknell.

"When you remove my femur, is there any chance you can look into or feel there to find out what's causing the necrotic mass in the back of my pelvis? I think my GYN doctor would be eternally grateful since that's been a big puzzle for him for a long time."

"We're not going in like Indiana Jones to explore," Dr. Bucknell promised. "But we'll look around and see what we can see."

My request for spinal anesthesia was agreed to, and I was alternately awake and asleep from tranquilizers during the surgery. From time to time I could hear the sound of an electric saw whirring through bone. Occasionally, I caught a glimpse of either Dr. Bucknell, Dr. Behrens, or one of the other assisting residents through my sedated eyes. I even tried to talk to the doctors while they worked. Now and then I saw Dr. Bucknell give a thumbs down sign, after which I would drift off to sleep again. I figured the anesthesiologist must have obliged him by giving me another shot of "shut-up medicine."

I emerged from slumber again just as the surgeons were winding down their procedure. "Was there any chance you found out what was in the back of my pelvis?" I asked Dr. Bucknell as he instructed his subordinates on closing the incision.

"Quite funny that you should ask," he teased. "This is what we found!" From behind the surgical screen Dr. Bucknell held up a bone with an extraterrestrial-looking mass at one end. The glob was purplish gray in color with veins coursing through it. It looked like something that had escaped from one of the *Alien* films.

"*What* is that thing?" I asked hesitatingly.

"That is the mass you had in the back of your pelvis," Dr. Bucknell responded matter-of-factly. "But I'll tell you all about it in the recovery room when you can remember."

A couple of hours later Dr. Bucknell visited me in the recovery room. He was still wearing his blood-spotted surgical greens. He explained that over the years pressure from the right femur head had worn a hole in the plastic acetabular cup in my pelvis which was installed during my hip replacement surgery in 1975.

Dr. Bucknell marked on my sheets with his ball-point pen to illustrate the position of the bones. The head of the femur actually had extended through the hole into my pelvic cavity and was causing scar tissue to form in the back of my pelvis.

"When we pulled your femur out of your pelvic cavity, it left a huge hole in your pelvis," Dr. Bucknell elaborated. "We had to sew surgical mesh over that opening in order to keep your intestines from dropping out of your pelvis. In time the mesh will heal over with muscle and tissue."

"Instead of being held together by baling wire and straw, I guess now we can add fish net as well," I joked.

In medical parlance, my recovery was unremarkable. Fortunately, due to the short time of the surgery, I avoided any infection complications.

There was little or no drainage from the incision, and, a couple of days later, Dr. Behrens pulled my drains.

Dr. Bucknell advised me that the main consequence of the surgery would be shrinkage of my leg, just as I had experienced on my left, because there was no bone to maintain its length.

Just prior to my discharge from the hospital, Dr. Behrens came by to bid me farewell.

"I guess I'm finished with you orthopods now," I joked.

"Not by a long shot, Mary. We're going to keep you on a short leash."

As we talked, it was clear that he was having trouble accepting my situation. "I had hopes that we could make you better, not worse," he confided, almost apologetically.

I looked at him gratefully as I extended my hand to say goodbye. "Believe me, Dr. Behrens, you have made me better!"

Ten days after surgery, I was released from the hospital, pale from blood loss, but otherwise feeling pretty well.

After a few outpatient sessions in physical therapy to help me learn to transfer more efficiently in my new condition, I returned to the Orthodedic Clinic for removal of my stitches.

"Sid Squid is here to have the stitches taken out," I jested when Dr. Behrens approached me with a suture-removing kit. My squid reference recalled his earlier prediction about my condition if I went through with having my femur removed.

Dr. Behrens, seemingly pleased by the appearance of my incision, quickly went about his task. As he was finishing up, I asked: "May I swim again?"

Taking my reference to sea animals a bit further, he replied: "Oh, sure. Just have Jack toss you in and let you flop around as best you can, not that you'll be able to go anywhere."

To the amazement of my doctors and probably a few other people, I'm still able to swim pretty well, if not up to par with my years in the Aqua Follies. Jack and I swim a quarter of a mile at least five times a week, year around. Surprisingly, I really don't need my legs to get me where I want to go.

The rest of 1988 was uneventful medically. However, in August we expanded our operatic horizons by attending four productions of the Santa Fe Opera, an event which would become an annual ritual for us.

Early in 1989 I started having problems with the scar on my left forearm where the chemotherapy drug had infiltrated my tissue back in 1974. I was experiencing some soreness, and the scarred area seemed to be spreading and getting more lumpy.

The dermatologists decided to do a punch biopsy at the site to rule out any renewal of malignancy. With a circular device about an eighth of an inch in diameter, a doctor pushed the instrument about a half inch into my arm and extracted some of the interior contents.

A week later the pathologist reported the sample to be necrotic tissue with no malignancy.

That was great news, of course. But it caused me to think "here we go again," recalling my long struggle attempting to find out what was causing necrotic tissue in my pelvis.

A month after the biopsy, the punch hole still had not healed. In fact, the wound looked the same as it did just after the procedure. Sensing a potential problem, Dr. Bucknell referred me to plastic surgery.

Dr. Morris was a tall, distinguished-looking man in his

mid-forties. When he examined my arm, he expressed surprise by the way the dermatologist had done the biopsy. "I'm sorry they did that," he stated. "When you punch into necrotic tissue, it doesn't heal."

Dr. Morris went on to outline several approaches for my situation, ranging from inserting a balloon-like device in my arm to stretch the skin, up to and including skin grafting.

As he talked I thought to myself that plastic surgeons apparently don't like to make anything relatively simple if it can be more complex.

Finally, I interjected a question. "Couldn't we just do a little cut, open it up, clean it out, and sew it back up again?"

"Well, yes," Dr. Morris acknowledged. "But I'm just not sure we can stretch your skin enough to close. If not, we may have to graft skin from another part of your body."

I agreed that would be all right.

A few days later I checked into the ENT/plastic surgery/specialties ward. Jack came along to help me take care of my preoperative work up.

While I waited for my chest X-ray, Jack returned to the ward to complete my paperwork. As he filled in the forms, the ward nurse, a male in his late thirties, discussed my case with Jack, who later told me of the conversation.

"How long has your wife been an invalid?" the nurse asked.

Jack was dumbfounded by the question. He stopped writing and looked up at the nurse. "Mary doesn't consider herself an invalid, and she doesn't think of people in wheelchairs as invalids," he said emphatically. "She's not a very combative person so she probably never would say anything. But believe me, she would certainly think a lot if you used that word in her presence."

The nurse seemed embarrassed. "I'm sorry. I didn't mean anything derogatory."

"She prefers terms like 'physically challenged' or something a little more modern than 'invalid,'" Jack added.

On the way to the cafeteria for lunch, Jack told me about his conversation with the nurse. Once inside the building, I said to him: "I'm going to roll over to our table, and you can wait on your invalid wife."

"Oh, no! You're going through the serving line with me so I don't have to hear that I've gotten you too much to eat."

Both of us had a good chuckle over that.

Later that day, the anesthesiologist came by to discuss my case. She explained that I would be getting a Bier block, which puts the arm to sleep but allows the patient to be awake.

"Do I bring the six pack or do you provide it?" I joked.

The next morning when I arrived in the operating room, the anesthesiologist was the first to greet me. "Where's your six pack?" she asked.

"Dr. Morris told me I couldn't bring it," I laughed.

I visited with Dr. Morris and the OR staff throughout the hour and a half surgery. Dr. Morris discovered there was adequate skin to close the incision, much to our collective relief.

"Are you sure you don't want to do a little nip and tuck elsewhere while I'm here?" I asked the doctor as the surgery was winding down.

"I'm afraid not," he replied. "The Army would drum me out before I was ready if I did that."

My recovery was uneventful, and I was released from the hospital after three days.

When I returned to the clinic ten days later to have the stitches removed, Dr. Morris was pleased with his handiwork. The necrotic tissue and scarring—a fifteen-year by-product of my struggle with cancer—had been removed. In its place was a thin, clean scar which would eventually become almost unnoticeable.

This was truly a new beginning for the rest of my life.

Chapter Forty

I arrived at the van repair shop just one minute before closing time.

When Bill, the shop foreman, saw my rear door open and my ramp extended outward, he shook his head and chuckled.

Bill could attest to the veracity of Jack's axiom: "To live by the wheel is to die by the wheel."

On more occasions than I care to remember, Bill has come to my rescue with an urgent repair to help me keep my independence.

After about an hour, Bill approached me in the waiting room: "Well, Mrs. Walker, we've got you fixed up one more time."

"What was wrong?"

"The weld was broken on one of the lift bars. When the relay hit it, the lift wouldn't work. Now you should be in good shape for awhile."

"I sure appreciate you working overtime," I assured him as I wished him a good weekend.

While driving home I thought, as I often do, that I was one lucky person.

The Fat Lady Hasn't Sung

Only a few years earlier, a person in my physical condition would have been relegated to the closet. But here I am today, driving my own vehicle and shopping alone.

I was reminded of the words of a little 90-year-old man at my mother's retirement home every time he sees me. "There are some people you just can't kill off," he always says, presumably with tongue in cheek.

I usually reply with "the fat lady hasn't sung," which is my shortened version of the now well-known expression, "the opera ain't over until the fat lady sings." My response usually elicits a hearty chuckle from the old-timer.

When I got home, Jack met me in the garage to help unload my groceries. "You're a little late," he observed. "Did you have any trouble?"

"Let's put the groceries away and get ready to go. I'll fill you in on the way to Houston."

An hour later we were driving toward Houston for our weekend with Placido.

Jack and I had been eagerly awaiting the Houston Grand Opera production of Verdi's *Otello* ever since it had been announced a year earlier. Not only has Jack convinced me that this work is Verdi's monumental masterpiece, but with Placido Domingo as the Moor, we were going to be able to see and hear this generation's foremost interpreter of the title role.

Francis Toye in 1931 asked himself a question Jack and I have asked ourselves many times: "Have the love, the passion, the anguish, and the hatred of human beings ever been presented to an audience with deeper insight or poignancy than in this music?"

Toye answers his own question. "I think not," he said. "Shakespeare himself did not do, could not have done, better."

We believe Toye was right!

Domingo himself—a conductor and musician of some note, in addition to possessing one of the finest dramatic tenor voices ever to sing this music—states that at the end of this opera he feels ". . .as if I have lived through the most tragically beautiful story ever told."

Otello's triumphant entrance in Act I is one of the most dramatic in all opera. As he comes down the gangway of his ship, he proclaims victory over the Turkish fleet. His first four notes are a magnificent one-word utterance of majestic power and beauty: "*Esultate!* [Rejoice!]."

As Domingo made his entrance in Houston and exclaimed "*Esultate!*" I glanced at Jack in the darkened opera house and silently moved my hand toward his. His eyes met mine as our hands joined simultaneously.

At that moment a thousand thoughts raced through my mind.

I thought "*Esultate!*" indeed—a thousand times "*Esultate!*"

I rejoice every day that I live for the life God has allowed me to continue.

I rejoice for the love and care my friends and neighbors have bestowed on me.

I rejoice for the love and help my parents, sister, children, and other members of my family have given me for so many years.

I rejoice for the professional care given so unstintingly for so long by a legion of health-care providers—doctors, nurses, corpsmen, aides, therapists, technicians, and administrators.

But most of all I rejoice for having Jack!

I must rephrase Toye's question. Have the love, the joy, the anguish, and the faithfulness between two human beings ever been experienced more fully and completely than between Jack and me?

I think not.

For over 35 years this wonderful man has stood by me—in sickness and in health—steadfastly faithful to his marital vows. Our love for each other continues to grow each year. He is truly my husband, my lover, and my best friend.

"*Esultate!*" indeed!

The fat lady hasn't sung for me!

Give the perfect gift to anyone whose life has been touched by cancer:

THE FAT LADY HASN'T SUNG

An Inspiring Story of Love, Hope and Triumph

BY MARY WALKER

ORDER FORM

Postal Orders: Hill Country Books, P.O. Box 791615-951
San Antonio, TX 78279-1615

Please send ____ copy/copies of *The Fat Lady Hasn't Sung* at $14.95 per copy.

Please send to:

Name: _____

Address: _____

City: _____ State: _____ Zip: _____

Sales tax:
   Please add 7.75% State sales tax for books shipped to Texas addresses.

Shipping:
   Book rate: $2.00 for the first book and 75 cents for each additional book.

   Priority mail: $4.00 per book.

Payment:
   ☐ Check
   ☐ Money Order